Emily's Walk

THE INDIANA AMUSEMENT PARK TRAGEDY
AND A FAMILY'S QUEST FOR JUSTICE

John Krull

Guild Press Emmis Publishing, LP

GUILD PRESS EMMIS PUBLISHING, LP
10655 Andrade Drive
Zionsville, Indiana 46077

ISBN: 1-57860-114-2

Library of Congress Catalog Number 2002107996

Cover photograph by Ernie Stigall

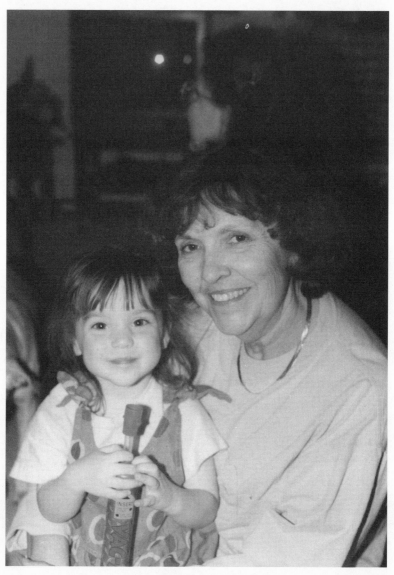

Emily with her Grandma, Nancy Jones.

To Nancy Jones, whose unending love
for her family helped guide them
through tragedy, and whose
eternal spirit can be seen as
the sparkle of hope in
her granddaughter's
eyes.

Acknowledgments

If you think of a story as a journey and a book as the vehicle that covers the ground, then you will realize a lot of people have a hand in building and maintaining that vehicle.

This book could not have been written without the contributions of many people. Doubtless, in offering thanks, I will forget someone. The oversight is not deliberate. It is just that the debts I accumulated in writing this book are so many in number that they are difficult to keep track of.

I am indebted to Bill Carr for his recommendations to improve the book, Tim Bender and Robin Babbitt for their legal counsel, Tom Pence for recommending this project to Emmis Publishing and to Emmis for helping to promote this book. I—and the Emily Hunt Foundation— also owe a tremendous debt of gratitude to the following people whose financial support helped get the book published: Jon and Katie Evans, Klipsch Audio Technologies, Hat World and the friends and family of Cindy Coers.

I am grateful to Florrie Binford Kichler for her generous and patient counsel, to Jim Denigan, Cathy Gibson, Susan Gray and Sidney Offit for their encouragement and criticism and to my publisher, Nancy Niblack Baxter, for patiently working with a first-time author in an unusual publishing arrangement.

I cannot thank enough the people who figure in this story and opened their lives to me during the reporting for this book: Ken Campbell, Ern Hudson, Candy Marendt, Jesse Villalpando, Luke Kenley and the staff of Gov. Frank O'Bannon.

Great as that gratitude is, it pales in comparison with the gratitude I owe to Bud Jones and his extended family for sharing so completely and so honestly the worst experience of their lives in the hope that it would make other lives better. The

Hunts—Emily, Nikki, Sarah, Amy and Mike—in particular have inspired me as they have so many others to face life's challenges with determination and grace.

My last debt is the most personal one. My daughter Erin, my son Ian and, most of all, my wife Jenny Labalme have shared this journey with me. Their love, support and patience inform every chapter, every page, every paragraph and every word.

John Krull
June, 2002

EMILY IN THE MORNING

Every school day, nine-year-old Emily Hunt's morning begins the same way.

Her father Mike opens the door to her bedroom at seven AM and says, "Good morning." Her three-year-old dog—a kinetic little part terrier, part Chihuahua mutt named Scooter—hops up onto Emily's specially designed hospital bed and licks her face.

"That's my good morning kiss," Emily says.

A dark-haired, dark-eyed girl with a shy smile that comes and goes as quickly as sunlight shimmering on the ripples of a pond, Emily lives her life on a schedule. Each day begins pretty much the same way because it has to—if she wants to live.

Right after she wakes up, she does a breathing treatment designed to strengthen her accident-weakened lungs. A machine designed to add air pressure to her lungs plugs into the tracheotomy tube in her throat.

Once that is done, her father dresses her and puts her in her wheelchair, the fourth such wheelchair she has had. She has lived in a wheelchair for more than half her life.

Some mornings she takes time to look around her room while she is taking her breathing treatment or her dad is dressing her.

Much of her room is like any other nine-year-old girl's. There are a couple of bookcases. The shelves are filled with knickknacks, stuffed animals, dolls, photos and inspirational sayings. Most of the stuffed animals and dolls are bears. A computer sits on her desk. A poster—a picture of dancing bears—hangs on one wall.

"I like bears," Emily says.

There are a few things one wouldn't expect to find in a nine-year-old girl's room. The hospital bed. A framed copy of a signed Indiana state law. And, on the wall right above the head of her bed, a beautiful painting of Emily in ballet garb, standing on point. The title of the painting is "Dreams of Dancing."

"That's my favorite thing in the room," Emily says.

Most mornings, though, Emily doesn't linger in her bedroom. She wheels out to the kitchen, and eats a quick breakfast—generally a strawberry Pop-Tart.

Three mornings a week, the bus picks her up to take her to school in Brownsburg. The other mornings, her mother drives her.

She knows when she leaves her home that her school day will be disrupted at least three and sometimes four times. She will be pulled out of class for different kinds of therapy, for medications and for other kinds of treatment.

In spite of the disruptions, she keeps her focus. She maintains a straight A record and loves reading and math, particularly.

There was a time, more than five years ago, when she did not have to sleep in a hospital bed—a time when she did not have to undergo constant sessions of physical therapy, occupational therapy and speech therapy, when she did not constantly have to take medication or subject herself to treatments. A time when she did not have to live in a wheelchair.

Back then, she had been a little girl like millions of other little girls. She ran instead of walked. She loved to play. And she dreamed of being a dancer.

If Emily resents being in a wheelchair, it does not show. But, then, it probably wouldn't. She is not the sort of little girl to show her feelings easily. Nor is she the sort to accept adversity as a permanent condition.

She takes pride in what to others might seem like small things. For a long time, she could not open the sliding glass door just off the kitchen of her family's home.

She worked with a strength coach, though, and gradually developed muscle enough to open the door. Now, whenever it is time for Scooter to go outside, Emily volunteers to open the door for him.

Emily does not remember the August Sunday that changed her life, nor her long stay in the hospital. She does not recall the desperate days when her parents feared that she would not live. She does not remember the pain—the agony— of having her jaw, collarbone and spine broken.

She only knows that her life was once one kind of journey, and now it is another kind.

The way her life changed is a story that needs to be told.

CHAPTER ONE

L ATER, LONG AFTER THE TRAIN HAD LEFT THE TRACKS AND carved such a deep hurt in his family, Bud Jones would remember the last moment when everything seemed right.

It was a cool August Sunday, late morning. All eight of Bud's grandchildren were close by, eager to have a good time at the amusement park he had chosen for a summer outing. Nancy, Bud's wife of nearly forty years, was seated in the train car just in front of him, with her arm around Emily, one of Bud's four-year-old twin granddaughters. Unlike her sister Nicole, who could be rambunctious, sometimes even aggressive, Emily was shy and sensitive, reticent. The other children loved rides, but not Emily. The treat for her on this Sunday was being with Grandma and Grandpa, not being at an amusement park.

To keep his granddaughter from being bored while they were waiting for the ride to start, Bud stretched out his hand and gave Emily's ponytail a tug. It was an old game for them, a way for Bud to tease her so that Grandma—Emily's favorite—could rush to her rescue. As soon as Bud let go of Emily's hair, she looked at him and smiled. Nancy shook her head in Bud's direction.

"No, no, Grandpa," Nancy said and laughed.

Bud laughed, too. Small moments like this gave him a feeling of comfort, a sense of closeness to his family. He thought that he and Nancy and Emily would have a few more minutes to play their little game. He would tug at his granddaughter's hair. She would pretend to be scared, and Nancy would feign reprimanding him. Everyone would have a few laughs on Grandpa.

Then the wheels started to turn, and the little train lurched forward. Almost immediately, Bud knew it was going too fast. Nancy turned toward him, a look of fear gripping her face.

It was the last time he saw her before the train wrecked, killing his wife and crippling his granddaughter.

The weekend that shattered Bud's family started as a kind of small celebration. Grandparents' weekend, the family called it. Two days of Bud and Nancy indulging the grandkids while their son and two daughters got a chance to spend some time alone with their spouses.

Bud and Nancy lived for weekends like this one. They saw them as a reward for working hard for forty years, for doing the constant labor and making the sacrifices necessary to raise and nurture a family. Just the year before, with the grandchildren in mind, they had bought a new house, a handsome stone home in a new subdivision on Indianapolis's west side. Most older couples look for a smaller home when their children start their lives. Not Bud and Nancy. They bought a home nearly twice as large as their old one, and furnished it to be a paradise for children. There was a small swimming pool in the backyard. Downstairs in the finished basement, Bud and Nancy had installed a wide-screen television set. A few yards away, in a video storage shelf, the happy grandparents stocked every children's movie Disney had released on VHS. Bud and Nancy wanted their home to be a place where their grandchildren came to feel happy, to know that they were loved and treasured.

Grandparents' weekend was the culmination of that devotion. When the children descended on Bud and Nancy's house Saturday morning, the grandparents divided them up by gender. The boys went fishing with Grandpa. The girls went shopping with Grandma.

After the fishing and the shopping, it was time for dinner. Bud took a certain amount of pride in spoiling his grandchildren. He loved to buy them the food their parents wouldn't. On previous grandparents' weekends, he had loaded all the kids into his car and driven them from fast-food place to fast-food place until each child got what he or she wanted. If that meant making stops at McDonald's, Taco Bell and Hardee's all on the same trip, so be it. In Bud's view, part of the joy of being a grandfather was finding ways to indulge his grandchildren. This time, he ordered three monster pizzas from a nearby Noble Roman's. By the time he got back from picking up the pies, the kids had changed into their swimsuits and were splashing wildly in the pool. Nancy watched them, a look resembling bliss on her face.

Nancy doted on her grandchildren. She called them her babies, and lived for opportunities to baby-sit. She and Emily— one of Amy's twin daughters—were particularly close. For some reason, Emily, an otherwise shy girl, had developed a fierce bond of affection with her grandmother. When Emily was just an infant—and in that difficult stage babies go through when they want to be handled only by their parents— the little girl still would allow her grandmother to pick her up and hold her. In fact, it went beyond that. Emily almost craved Nancy's presence. Whenever Nancy and Emily were together, regardless of who else was present, the little girl demanded that her grandmother hold her. Nancy toted her around while Emily clung to her grandmother's neck. Other members of the family actually made a joke out of it. "Grandma's goiter," they called Emily, or "G.G.," for short.

That Saturday night, Emily didn't cling quite so closely to her grandmother. With all her other cousins around, she was busy playing. Like the other kids, she jumped and splashed in the pool. When Bud showed up with the three huge pizzas, all of the children rushed forward to grab the thick slices of pepperoni pie.

Later, after the children had been fed and bathed, Bud and Nancy herded them down to the basement. While their grandchildren arranged their sleeping bags, Nancy picked out a Disney video to pop into the VCR. Not more than fifteen minutes after the movie started, every child in the room was sound asleep.

As Bud checked to make sure the children were snug in their sleeping bags and turned out the lights, he heard Nancy putting away dishes and other debris from the day's activities. The sight of the children sleeping and his wife, their grandmother, moving one flight above them comforted him.

Not for the first time in his life, he thought his family had been blessed.

The next morning, Bud and Nancy awoke early. They got cleaned up, put some coffee on and enjoyed a couple of minutes to themselves before the children got up.

Much as he loved his family, Bud treasured moments alone with Nancy. Even though they had been married for thirty-nine years—and together, really, for more than forty-five—he still got a thrill from seeing her. She was a woman who took great care with her appearance. Even when she only meant to spend the day working around the house, she wore a sweat suit that was color-coordinated with her shoes and the band she wore in her hair. When he came home after work, Nancy always was nicely put together. She made the end of the day a thing for him to look forward to. The touch of her hand reached some secret spot in him and made him feel a little more alive. He had heard that many married couples settled into a kind of companionship that was more emotional than sexual. He and Nancy had a strong emotional bond, to be sure. She was his best friend. But he still felt a powerful physical need for her, a strong desire to be close to her.

Once they entered their teen years, his children had started teasing him and Nancy about it. Whenever he reached out to pat his wife on her rear or kiss the back of her neck, one of the children would laugh and say, "We better watch Mom and Dad. They're getting frisky again." The teasing, Bud understood, had been born of a kind of satisfaction. Seeing their parents so obviously in love gave his children a sense of security, and made them believe that little could harm them. Their parents' love was like a protective shield around the family.

As Bud and Nancy puttered around the upstairs making coffee and getting ready for the day, the grandchildren began to awaken downstairs. That was the way it always happened on these weekends. First one child would open an eye, then another. Within fifteen minutes, all of them would be up, eager to have breakfast and another day of fun with Grandma and Grandpa.

Bud grabbed a couple of the boys to go buy doughnuts from a nearby Roselyn's Bakery while Nancy put the other children to work preparing picnic lunches for the trip up to the Old Indiana Family Fun-n-Water Park, an amusement park just outside Thorntown, Indiana. Bud liked taking the kids to the park. Only a forty-five-minute drive from his house, it was close enough to be a convenient day trip. Old Indiana also was less intimidating to small children than large amusement parks like Kings Island or Six Flags. The rides were smaller and, Bud thought, probably safer. The grounds also were smaller, which meant the job of keeping track of a group of over-stimulated children would be easier than at a larger place.

This wasn't to be a solo trip. Bud's sister Polly had charge of her grandchildren, too, and would be going up to the park with the Joneses. The plan was for everyone to drive up together in one large caravan, but Polly called mid-morning while Bud's grandchildren still were working their way through their doughnuts to stay that her brood was just too restless to sit still. She was going to load them all into the car and take off for Old Indiana, she said. She would see Bud and Nancy at the park.

After the call, Bud and Nancy got the grandchildren organized. They packed the trunks of their two cars with picnic baskets and coolers filled with soda pop. They separated the children into two groups—one set for Grandpa's car, another for Grandma's. Just before they left the house, Bud gave Nancy a quick goodbye kiss.

On the drive north to Old Indiana, Bud kept the kids occupied with car games. They competed to see who could spot the most out-of-state license plates and who could see the most American flags. In no time, the drive to the park went by, and Bud and Nancy found themselves unloading the cars while the children urged them to hurry up, hurry up.

It was 11:15 AM, August 11, 1996. Polly was already there. Once Bud and Nancy got their eight grandchildren into the park, she came up to say hello. There wasn't much time for chitchat, because the kids were eager to play. Half of Bud's grandchildren wanted to go get in line for the log chute, a ride that resembled a roller coaster with water.

The other half, the younger kids, were eager to go play in Kiddi-Land. Bud told Nancy and Polly that he would take the little ones, including the twins Emily and Nicole, over to Kiddi-Land. Everyone got in line for the boats, a slow ride that wouldn't be too frightening for children. All the kids wanted to do the helicopters, their favorite ride, first. Bud told them that they could do the helicopters next.

The boat ride didn't take long. Before it ended, Polly and Nancy came walking over. The children clambered off, and Bud began herding them over to the helicopters. Even though it was early August, a chill gripped the air. Polly said she was cold and that a cup of coffee sure would feel good. On the way to the helicopters, they walked by a concession stand. No coffee. The adults joked that they would just have to tough it out without something warm to drink. Bud arranged the children in the helicopters and watched them take off.

He found himself on the opposite side of the gate from Nancy. He looked at his wife and smiled. She smiled back. Bud thought that his wife was a remarkably pretty woman.

The kids climbed out of the helicopter, energized by the spin in the air. They were eager to do more rides. In quick succession, they did the Kiddi-Roller Coaster and the horse and cart ride. After the roller coaster, the kids thought the horse and cart ride was boring. They wanted something a little more noisy, a mechanical ride.

The miniature train seemed to be just the ticket. It was a small train, designed to run at about eight miles per hour over a short, winding track through the woods. The cars were no taller than an adult's hips and the winding track covered only a few hundred yards of rails. Bud had taken the kids on the ride before, and they had always had a good time.

When they got to the entrance gate for the train ride, Bud thought something was wrong. The attendant, a young man in his late teens, had his back turned toward the crowd. He didn't seem interested in who got on the ride and who didn't. Others in the crowd started to duck under the rope, so Bud, Nancy, Polly and the children followed suit.

Most of the children found seats in the first passenger car. Nancy and Emily took spots in the last row of that first car. Bud grabbed the first seat in the second car. Polly sat behind him.

While they waited for the ride to begin, Bud reached forward to pull Emily's ponytail. His granddaughter smiled. Nancy laughed and said, "No, no, Grandpa."

Bud began thinking about teasing Emily some more when the train lurched forward. Almost immediately, he realized the train was going too fast. It rocked from side to side, and seemed to barrel along the tracks.

Nancy turned toward him. The look on her face begged him to do something to slow the train down.

The little train shot over a small bridge spanning a tiny

pond and came to a curve. A little stand of trees stood off to the side, next to a gentle embankment that sloped about fifteen feet down to a chain-link fence. Bud was just about to try to signal the driver to slow down when the train flipped over.

The wreck threw Bud feet first down the slope. He hit the ground less than ten feet from the train, but he was moving so fast when he landed that his left leg broke when he hit the earth. The bone midway down his shin just snapped. Even as his leg broke, Bud didn't think that the accident was dangerous. He worried that having the train jump the tracks would scare the children and make them not want to do any more rides.

Within an instant, a greater fear crowded that worry out of his mind. Out of the corner of his eye, he saw something that chilled him. Nancy had been hurled against a slender tree at full-speed. He had not seen the impact, but he could see her body sliding down the tree trunk. She landed in a heap, her limbs akimbo.

Bud could not be sure of what he saw or felt. Shock began to set in almost immediately. Sights came to him in shades of gray. Sounds were muffled, as if they had been muted.

When he stopped sliding, he first saw his grandchildren Sarah and Drew. They had been thrown up against the fence a few yards ahead of him. They weren't moving. Bud started to drag himself by his hands and elbows toward them when he heard his sister yell that he should get to Nancy and Emily. Polly said it looked like they were seriously hurt.

Bud dragged himself over to his wife's side. Even though he was less than ten feet away from Nancy, crawling over to her side was torturous and seemed to take forever. The ground gave way under his elbows and hands. What he found when he got to Nancy was not encouraging. Being thrown against the tree had mangled her. Her face was battered, bloody and almost unrecognizable. The bark on the tree had been broken off where her head had hit and there was blood on the wood. His wife's blood.

Emily had fallen beside her. The little girl was on her back. Blood trickled from her mouth. Bud couldn't tell if his granddaughter was breathing, so he started to massage her stomach. Her arm looked as if it had been wrenched out of its socket. He started to move it and Emily grimaced. He knew then that she was alive but badly injured.

He elbow-dragged himself back to Nancy. Blood gurgled from her mouth. Bud tried to force his wife's mouth open so she wouldn't drown in her own blood, but it seemed hopeless. He touched her leg and realized that Nancy was losing body temperature.

A thought cut through the shock: His wife was dying and there was nothing he could do about it.

The train's engine and several cars were lying on the ground just beyond the little brook. Tipped over on the ground, the train cars looked ridiculously small—too tiny to do much damage, Bud tried to convince himself.

He looked up. Sarah and Drew somehow had collected themselves. They were walking toward him. They were holding hands, just as they had been taught to do in an emergency. Both children were crying.

Sarah saw him and said, "Grandpa, I don't want to ride any more rides today."

Bud looked at his granddaughter and said, "OK, we won't."

Then he began to yell for someone to help his family.

CHAPTER TWO

IT SEEMED TO BUD THAT HELP WAS A LONG TIME IN COMING. AS he lay there beside the slender tree, his bloodied wife and granddaughter alongside him, minutes, even hours, seemed to tick away.

He was in shock. His broken leg had not even begun to hurt yet. He knew something was wrong with his thoughts. Everything he saw—the boundary fence, the little tree, his grandchildren, even his wife—seemed to be distorted by a gray filminess, almost as if all the things and people around him were wrapped in gauze.

There would be stray instants, though, when he would see everything around him with a terrifying clarity. He would look at his wife and know that she was dying. He would see Emily and know that she was hurt bad. Maybe she was dying, too. And he would know that, with his broken leg unable to support his weight, there was nothing he could do to help them.

At those times, panic rose in him like a skittish animal. He felt a helplessness that crowded out every other sensation. His loved ones were hurt and dying beside him. Moments ticked by with him powerless to help either Nancy or Emily. Where were the police, the medics? Why didn't someone come?

He felt the presence of someone standing near him, almost over him. It was the teenager who had been driving the train, the one Bud had been ready to signal to slow down just before the accident happened. Trembling, the boy looked down at Bud.

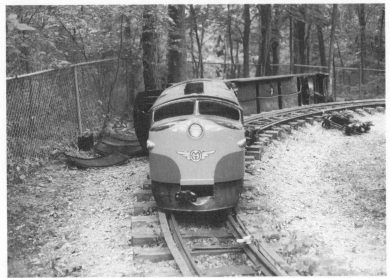

The minature train that jumped the tracks sits idle at the Old Indiana Family Fun-n-Water Park. Note the turned-over car near the tree that Nancy and Emily hit.

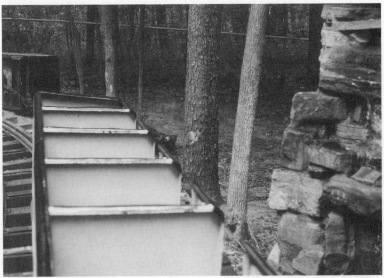

This is a rear-view photo of the train. Note the impact on the tree.

"Man, what in the hell were you thinking?" Bud asked, his voice shaking.

"I wasn't going too fast," the boy answered.

Bud felt a rage build in him. If the boy hadn't been driving too fast, why were Nancy and Emily lying in heaps beside him? Why were they lying there, dying, while Bud waited for help?

"Yes, you were," Bud spat back.

"No, I wasn't," the boy said, less confidently this time.

"You were," Bud said.

Other people started to gather around Bud. They wanted to find him a stretcher or build makeshift splints for his leg. He couldn't understand why they were focusing their attention on him.

"I'm fine," he said. They wouldn't leave him alone. Couldn't they see that Nancy and Emily needed to be taken care of first? Couldn't they understand that? How long would it take for someone professional, someone who could really help, to show up?

"Help my wife," Bud barked as people continued to fuss over him. "Help my granddaughter. Take care of them first."

A woman came to take charge. She demanded that body boards be brought to the scene immediately. She walked over to the boundary fence and tore out a section of it.

The people helping tended to Emily first. They placed a neck collar on her and put her on one of the body boards. Bud was glad that his granddaughter was getting aid. He just hoped that these people knew what they were doing. Where were the cops?

Bud saw a man put a neck collar on Nancy. The man cradled Nancy's head in his lap and felt for a pulse. As he watched the man work, Bud listened closely, hoping to hear some words of encouragement. The man didn't say anything.

Within moments, the woman had brought the section of fence over to Nancy. Together she and the man lifted Nancy on to the fence to carry away. Bud felt something sink within him. Nancy wasn't moving, and hope fled from him like water evaporating. As they lifted her, Bud put his hand on his wife's leg. It was cold to the touch.

In truth, help had not been long in coming.

The little train left the tracks at the Old Indiana Family Fun-n-Water Park at about ten minutes 'til noon. Boone County Sheriff Ern K. Hudson got the call at 11:57. He was only four miles from the park at the time, in the police cruiser with his wife, Judy, who also was a captain with the sheriff's department. He drove fast. The speedometer jumped to over ninety miles per hour while the car screamed over the country roads leading through rural Boone County to Old Indiana. He pulled into the gate just as the clock was striking noon.

Over the years, a lot of people had underestimated Ern Hudson. A big, fleshy man with a hefty paunch, a wide face and thinning hair, Ern moved slowly and talked even more slowly. On this day, because it was summer, he was wearing one of the bright red T-shirts that Boone County Sheriff's Department officers wore on summer days. When he turned his head, the flesh around his neck folded up. Even on cool days, sweat dripped down his forehead.

Nor did he talk like a particularly formidable man. At its best, Ern Hudson's brand of conversation was earthy and unrefined. At its worst, it was salty, even vulgar. Ern Hudson was not the kind of guy who fit in easily at highbrow country clubs. He did not belong in a boardroom. He was not fancy or sophisticated. He took pride, in fact, in being none of those things—in being a good old boy who bulled his way through until he had done what needed to be done. He let others worry about working angles. Ern's style was to sink into something and hold on until the bitter end, to maintain his grip until the truth stopped squirming.

When he got to the train tracks, the sheriff realized this was no minor accident. He tried to control the crowd that was gathering. He moved people back and did his best to find out what had happened. The damage, he quickly learned, was significant.

At least ten people had been hurt when the train wrecked. It looked like at least two of the victims—a middle-aged woman and a little girl—had life-threatening injuries. Everyone was panicked and angry. It helped that rescue teams of medics had arrived, and that two emergency helicopters had been called for the woman and the little girl. He knew their names now. Nancy Jones and Emily Hunt.

Ern realized he needed someone skilled in accident reconstruction to determine what went wrong. He called for his best accident investigator, a sheriff department's lieutenant named Ken Campbell.

Campbell got to the park quickly. He knew Old Indiana well. For several years, he and several other deputies had earned some extra money by moonlighting as security guards at the park.

A fit man of middling height, Campbell made a sharp contrast with his boss, the sheriff. Ern was a backslapper, a naturally friendly man at home swapping stories with his buddies on a small-town sidewalk. Campbell was more laconic, less willing or able to project his personality.

One quality the two men shared was doggedness. Campbell believed in thoroughness. The repetitiveness—asking the same questions again and again, staring at the same sights over and over—that drove other men crazy merely intrigued him. The challenge for him in an investigation was in putting the pieces together, finding out why the car started to slide and what speed it was going before the driver hit the brakes.

He set to work on solving this puzzle right away. He approached Carl Verh, the park's assistant general manager, and asked to see the train's maintenance records. Verh told Campbell that someone would bring the records right over.

The next logical step was to interview the driver. He found the driver, a scared and shaken young man by the name of

Jamie Marquess, and took him over to a nearby building so they could talk privately. Marquess, Campbell quickly learned, was little more than a kid, a twenty-three-year-old who looked much younger than his years. The young man was afraid that he would lose his job for saying the wrong thing. And he was terrified that he'd never find another steady paycheck. Campbell had Marquess take drug and alcohol tests. He found that the young man had been sober when the train wrecked.

Campbell asked the young man what happened. A disjointed story emerged as Marquess answered questions.

The young man said that he had given the train some gas to get it started. The train started wobbling as it came down the little hill. He tried to brake, but couldn't slow the train down. Then the train started to tip, and the cars fell over.

Campbell asked if the train had been running well. Marquess said yes, but that the engines were not operating "at one-hundred percent." He explained that the train had had a history of problems, including engine, brake and derailer breakdowns. The maintenance staff knew about the problems.

"The train always has something wrong," Marquess said.

Campbell decided it was time to have another talk with Carl Verh. Enough time had gone by for Verh to have put together the train's maintenance records. The records would tell Campbell if Marquess was telling the truth or trying to come up with an excuse for causing the accident.

As Campbell headed back to the accident site, he asked Verh again and again for the records. Verh smiled and said the papers were on their way. People were collecting them and copying them at just that moment, Verh said.

Campbell walked around the train track. What he saw appalled him. He found pieces of the train—derailers, brakes and other parts—far from the scene of the wreck. Pieces must have been falling off it for days, weeks or even months before it jumped the tracks.

He walked back to Verh and demanded the records. Verh told him that he had assembled the maintenance records, but said the park's insurance company had told him not to hand them over.

Campbell walked away from the exchange convinced that Verh and Old Indiana were trying to hide something. He talked with the sheriff about it. Ern shook his head.

It had been Ern's experience that people started lying to cops when they had done something pretty damn bad.

While Ern Hudson and Ken Campbell tried to figure out what had happened at Old Indiana, rescue workers loaded Bud Jones into an ambulance to make the forty-minute trip to Methodist Hospital in Indianapolis.

His sister Polly had insisted that the rescue teams carry them to Methodist. Bud had pushed for the hospital, too. They knew that Methodist had emergency helicopters—Lifelines, they were called. The air rescue would get Nancy and Emily to the hospital fast.

That was all Bud could think about. He tried to convince himself that his wife and granddaughter really hadn't looked that bad. Perhaps their injuries weren't as severe as he thought they were. Maybe they would be okay, after all.

As soon as those thoughts appeared, others crowded them out. The picture of his wife crumpled beside the tree, blood running out of her mouth, stood out vividly. He could see his granddaughter beside her, her arm twisted at an odd angle, her tiny body broken on the ground. He could see his other grandchildren in tears, his sister frantic to see that everyone was cared for.

Before the ambulance left the park, Polly had started calling the family members who were at Old Indiana. The others would want to know how bad things were. Besides, with both Bud and Nancy seriously hurt, Polly would need help with the children.

Bud's son, David, had been the first to arrive. He had driven from his home in a suburb north and east of Indianapolis to Old Indiana at more than 100 miles per hour to get there.

He had seen both Nancy and Emily while they waited for the helicopters to arrive. He had seen his mother, battered and bloodied.

As Bud was being loaded into the ambulance, David had rushed up and thrown his arm around his father. David hugged Bud so hard that it hurt. For a long moment, David just sobbed on his father's chest, as if he were still a boy and his father could make everything right again.

But Bud couldn't make everything right again. As he lay flat on his back on a stretcher in the ambulance, he thought of his family. His wife, her face crushed. His granddaughter, her arm and God knows what else broken. His other grandchildren, terrified. Polly, overwhelmed. David, sobbing. All of them in pain. All of them frightened.

"And it's all my fault," Bud couldn't help thinking.

He had picked the park and made the plans, he thought. He had led them onto the train. He had ignored his doubts about the rickety tracks and the inattentive driver. As the father and grandfather, he believed, it was his duty to protect his wife and take care of the young ones. They were all hurt, maybe dying. It was hard not to feel that he had failed to do his job as a man. A suffocating feeling of responsibility fell on him like a huge mound of dirt.

The ambulance shook and jostled as it moved over the bumpy roads leading away from the park. The attendant apologized for the rough roads. From up front, a radio blared, keeping the drivers in contact with the hospital. Bud could hear the hospital dispatcher giving the helicopters directions to get to the park. The copters were close; they would be landing and picking up Nancy and Emily in just a moment.

Then Bud heard the dispatcher tell one of the helicopter pilots to return to the hospital. Only one of accident victims, a little girl, still needed help.

That was how Bud learned that his wife of thirty-nine years had died.

He closed his eyes and shook his head, and wished he

could make the day march backward.

At Old Indiana, Ern Hudson and Ken Campbell found the scope of the accident widening before them like the mouth of a river.

The train wreck had injured eight people. One of them—a woman whose name, they learned, was Nancy Jones—already was dead. A little girl had been seriously hurt, too. Her name was Emily Hunt. The medics told Ern and Ken not to bet on her recovery. It appeared that the little girl's spine had been fractured. Children that young and that small generally didn't survive injuries that severe. An older man, Bud Jones, the dead woman's husband, had suffered a broken leg. Another older woman, Pauline Gentry, had broken her arm. Several other children had suffered bruises and cuts.

It was hard to believe that one little train—a kiddie ride at an amusement park—could cause so much misery. But it had. And there was nothing to do now but figure out what had happened, find out why the train had left the tracks. The job wouldn't be an easy one, because it looked like the Old Indiana owners already were trying to cover their trail. Attention to detail would be even more important than it normally was. Campbell realized that he had to photograph and study every section of the train and every foot of the track. And he had to do it before anyone had a chance to alter the evidence.

As he walked along the accident site, Campbell saw a man pick up a man's shoe near the spot where Bud Jones had landed after being thrown out of the train car. Campbell couldn't believe it. He assumed that the man had to be an Old Indiana employee.

"Hey, don't touch that!" Campbell yelled in his best tough-cop voice. "That's evidence!"

The man surprised Campbell. Instead of apologizing and putting the shoe down, the man flared back.

"This belongs to my father!" he shouted.

Campbell apologized, and expressed his condolences. That was the way Ken Campbell met David Jones. David had just finished identifying his mother's body.

Bud's hospital room and the waiting room buzzed with activity.

Word of the wreck had circulated, and all the family members and friends were beginning to gather at Methodist. Bud kept asking about Emily, but the answers he got from the doctors and nurses were guarded, even evasive. They kept saying that Bud needed to focus on healing himself, that he needed to rest.

They didn't understand, Bud thought, how hard it was for a man to rest when he knew his wife was dead and his entire family was battered.

Finally, the nurses began to let family members in to see him. Bud gathered from his children that Emily's condition wasn't good—that there was a better than even chance that she wouldn't live.

The news crushed Bud. He felt worse than hurt. He felt incomplete. Nancy, he thought, would know how to help him with this. Nancy would help him take care of his family. She always had. But Nancy was gone, and Bud didn't know what to do.

He cursed himself. He replayed the accident again and again in his mind. He heard Nancy saying, "No, no, Grandpa," after he tugged on Emily's pigtail. He saw Emily's shy smile. He felt the train start, then pick up speed. He saw Nancy turn toward him, her face begging him to stop the train. He felt himself thrown out of the car, and saw, once more, Nancy's body slide down the tree. He felt the earth beneath him as he crawled toward Nancy and Emily and saw, again, Emily grimace as he moved her arm.

Bud looked up to see his latest visitor. It was the one person he almost dreaded confronting, his daughter Amy's husband. Emily's father. The man who had trusted him to take care of his little girl. Mike Hunt.

"Oh God, Mike, I'm so sorry. I'm so sorry. So sorry," Bud said, his voice almost failing.

The tears started to crawl down his cheeks.

Mike reached out and patted Bud on the hand.

"What do you mean, Bud? Don't be ridiculous. This wasn't your fault. You didn't have anything to do with this," Mike said.

Bud couldn't hear it. He shook his head, then looked up at his son-in-law.

"Please, Mike," he said. "Can you ever forgive me? Please, you've got to forgive me. Please forgive me."

CHAPTER THREE

Mike Hunt saw grandparents' weekend not just as an opportunity for Bud and Nancy to spend some time with their grandchildren, but as an opportunity for him and Amy to spend a little bit of time together. With three children in the house—all of them bright, energetic girls under the age of six—finding time to be a husband and wife rather than a father and mother wasn't easy.

Not that he minded. In a way, it almost surprised Mike that he had been so ready to be a father. Until he met Amy, he had not been the sort of guy who could commit himself easily. He had grown up as part of a large family in a suburb of Denver. As a child and teenager, he had been a good enough student—top ten percent of his class—but his real love had been sports. Stocky and surprisingly fast for someone as heavily muscled as he was, he had played football and baseball in high school. He had started out playing fullback on the freshman team, but the varsity needed offensive linemen. As fullback he'd never be more than a reserve, but being on the line meant a chance to play every game. He started almost living in the weight room, pumping iron until he had bulked up to 185 pounds—pretty sturdy for a guy 5 feet 8 inches tall.

Football, he learned, was a game of leverage. He found that he could hold his ground and even beat guys much bigger than he was by finding the right spot to shove against. It was knowing where to hit that mattered. Even a little guy could come out on top if he used his weight in the right way.

Baseball came to him much more easily. He played centerfield, and played it well enough to attract the attention of the coaches at the state's best college baseball team, Northern Colorado University. Winning their attention, though, was easier than getting playing time. He sat on the bench for one year, then two. He hurt his knee sliding into base one day. By the time the injury had healed, he had decided that he'd had enough of watching games from the dugout. He quit the team.

To fill his time, he took up rodeo. He rode bulls for two years, traveling around Colorado, waiting for the gate to open so the bull could come exploding out of the shute with him holding on for dear life. Bull-riding, Mike found, gave a man a keen sense of focus. Eight seconds did not seem like a long time to the people sitting in the stands. For the man on the back of the bull, though, it could be an eternity, a seemingly endless stretch of time in which something, anything, could go horribly wrong. To keep disaster at bay, a rodeo rider had to keep his mind clear and sharp so he could concentrate on the essentials. It was easy to be distracted by things that seemed to be dangers but really weren't. Having the bull's horns jerking and jabbing just a few feet away from the rider's chest and abdomen appeared to be a threat, but the horns weren't the danger. As long as a man stayed on the bull, there was no way the horns could reach him. The bull's legs were the things that could hurt him. Once the rider got thrown, he could be stomped by the bull, then gored at the bull's leisure. Staying on the bull took more than strength; it took presence of mind. A good rider had to be able to sense where the bull was going and shift his own weight accordingly. Mike was pretty good at rodeo.

He graduated from Northern Colorado with a degree in finance and economics in 1985. He finished third in his class. Normally, that would have guaranteed him a good job somewhere in the state, but that was a hard year for Colorado. The oil industry had gone soft, and the state's fortunes had plunged. All over Denver there were abandoned and vacant office buildings.

Rather than look for jobs that didn't exist, Mike decided to buy time and continue his education. Notre Dame University had a special MBA program that could be completed in a year. He applied, and was accepted.

That meant moving to South Bend, Indiana, but he was eager to see some other parts of the country before he settled down. The year at Notre Dame passed quickly. The first month was an intensive study program, a kind of intellectual boot camp for graduate students hoping for careers in business. He and his classmates got up every morning, attended classes, then studied together right up until they tumbled into bed for a couple of hours of sleep. The next morning, they started all over again. That first month of graduate school taught him a lot about working under deadline pressure and about thinking clearly even when he was exhausted.

When he finished at Notre Dame in 1986, finding a job wasn't difficult for a guy with an MBA. At a big school like that, the companies came offering jobs. He found a good one with Oxford Real Estate, a company that managed apartment complexes. They wanted him to move to Indianapolis, about three hours south of South Bend. It was a sweet deal for a guy still only twenty-three years old. They offered him a lot of money and the opportunity to live at a discounted rent in one of the company's best apartments. What more could a young man want?

He moved to Indianapolis in the late summer of 1986. Less than a year later, he met Amy.

At first, Amy didn't want to go out with Mike. Didn't want to meet him, in fact.

Her childhood friend, Cheryl Broadstreet, worked for him. Amy had known Cheryl ever since they both were in elementary school on the west side of Indianapolis. They were close, almost like sisters. Because Amy had been the baby in her family, she never had felt like a full partner with her older brother David and sister Kathy. They were the older kids and she was the little one, the tag-along who had to be looked after. Perhaps that was one of the reasons Cheryl's friendship had meant so much to her. It was nice to have someone close who was the same age and didn't treat her like a little kid.

Still, that didn't mean Amy had to take Cheryl's advice when it came to romance. Even though she was only in her early twenties at the time, Amy knew that finding a life partner would not be an easy task for her. Around the dinner table and in a thousand other ways, Bud and Nancy had emphasized the importance of family and the obligations being part of a family imposed. An attractive young woman with blonde hair and her mother's big round eyes, Amy had been asked out often since she started dating. She generally lost interest pretty quickly, though, because almost inevitably the man was the product of a fractured home or a family that didn't take responsibility as seriously as hers did. Amy could not imagine having another kind of marriage or home than the sort her parents did. If she couldn't have that, then she didn't want it at all.

What Amy heard from Cheryl about Mike wasn't particularly reassuring. Even though Cheryl tried to put her boss in the best light possible, Amy figured out that he was a guy who spent a lot of time working, devoted much of his free time to hanging out with friends in town, and did a lot of traveling on weekends to visit still more buddies who were scattered around the country.

All of that sounded unconventional and even a little unreliable to Amy. It sure didn't sound like a guy who was eager to settle down and ready to assume the responsibilities of having a family. Amy did not know much about the world outside Indiana. Born and raised in Indianapolis, she had gone to high school there and traveled all of sixty miles to go to college at Ball State University in Muncie. When she graduated four years later, with a degree in elementary education, she came back to her hometown to teach in the Indianapolis Public Schools. The only trips of any duration she had taken outside the state were the annual vacations to Florida she went on with her parents.

Cheryl was persistent. She kept after Amy, and Amy knew her friend was pestering Mike, too. Finally, Amy agreed to meet him. Cheryl said Mike was going to call her. No, Amy said. She didn't want to have to make small talk over the phone with someone she didn't even know. Couldn't they just meet somewhere as part of a group and then see if they had anything in common?

Cheryl worked out the details. She talked to Mike and found out he would be at a nighclub on the north side of the city, with a buddy who was visiting from out of town. That didn't sound promising, but Amy went anyway.

She was surprised. Mike didn't seem like the other guys she had met. He was friendly and down-to-earth, the kind of man who seemed secure about himself. From the moment she met him, she felt comfortable with him.

They danced that night, and talked, sketching out their life stories. The details could be filled in later, she figured. When she and Cheryl got ready to leave, Mike asked Amy for her number.

He called the next day to ask her if she wanted to have dinner and see a movie with him. They went out that night.

In an odd way, Amy's initial worries about Mike were right.

Until he met her, he had never really had a girlfriend. In college he had dated women, but rarely for very long. After three or four weeks, he would start to feel claustrophobic and begin to hunger for open space. He owned a motorcycle then. When things started to feel too close and smothering, he would twist the throttle back and head up into the mountains—without telling the woman he was involved with where he was going. When he came back, the woman rarely was in a forgiving or understanding mood.

With Amy it was different. Something about her just seemed to fit. Because her family had lived on a tight budget when she was growing up, there was a lot of life she had not seen. Mike had been around people who were jaded, who took life's pleasures for granted. Amy was the opposite of that. When he took her out to a nice restaurant or they went to spend a weekend in the Smoky Mountains or Chicago, she was enthusiastic in a way that went beyond mere appreciation. She took almost a child's glee in discovering new things, in seeing what the world could offer. Watching Amy enjoy herself so much left Mike with a feeling of warmth that surprised him.

For Amy, the dates and the trips were nice, but they weren't what drew her to Mike. She felt that they shared the same values, that they looked at life in the same way. Like her, he came from a close-knit family. He was the fourth of Bob and Kay Hunt's six children. In the Hunt family, as in the Jones family, the dinner hour was sacred. No one missed it. The difference was in the tone. For the Joneses, dinner was a time to recount the day's events and thrash out any family problems. The Hunts, on the other hand, were teasers. As soon as the plates hit the table, the jokes started. Someone was always on the hot seat.

The families were similar in other ways, too. Mike's mother also stayed home to raise her children. Like Bud Jones, Bob Hunt started with little, worked hard and gradually began to make a good living. He developed a multiple-listing real estate book that he marketed on his own, and eventually did well with it. But the first years of his new business were difficult. There were a lot of days Mike could remember when his father would work all day, come home for dinner with the family, then head back to the office in the evening. The lesson took. Mike came to believe that almost any dream could become real if a person pursued it hard enough.

The family imparted other lessons as well. Each morning when the children got up, they found a list of chores their mother had prepared waiting for them. They had to do the jobs Kay had given them before they could get ready for school or go out to play. The message was clear. Work came first.

That was how Mike pursued his career. He figured he should establish himself before got married and had a family of his own. He wanted to be free to go into the office whenever he needed to or to pursue any opportunity that presented itself regardless of where the opportunity presented itself.

His commitment to his career almost ended his courtship with Amy. After they had dated for more than a year, Mike's company offered him a promotion. The catch was that he had to move to Los Angeles.

He took the job, and he and Amy talked about trying to maintain a long-distance relationship. Without a commitment, she didn't see how it would work. He didn't think he was ready to get married. When he left Indianapolis, they promised to stay in contact, but there was no understanding between them.

The job in Los Angeles was a young man's dream. It involved scouting out good sites for building and helping supervise construction. Mike spent entire days traveling up and down the coast, tramping over choice pieces of land. He was outdoors a lot, which suited him.

Something was missing, though. More and more it seemed to him that the part of his life that was missing was Amy.

He came to Indianapolis for a real estate seminar in November, and he and Amy got together. After Mike had moved to California, the two of them had fallen into the habit of calling each other once a month or so to check in. They had avoided talking about where their relationship was going, what possibilities they had together.

When they met for dinner, Mike asked Amy to come visit him in California. She started to refuse, began to say that it made no sense for her to do that unless they planned to get married. He stopped her and said that he really wanted her to come visit him. She knew then, just from listening to his voice and looking at him, that he had made his decision. She said she would come see him.

She came out on her spring break from teaching. They

had talked more often since his November visit, and had begun to clarify their relationship. They spoke of the future, and of the kind of family they would like to have. Both of them knew, without it ever being really said, that they would be engaged before Amy got on the plane to go home. The anticipation did not make the moment any less sweet.

Mike asked Amy to marry him only hours after she had arrived in Los Angeles. It was time. They began to plan their wedding. They were both twenty-six and ready to begin their lives together. They would have to marry in a hurry, because Amy would need at least part of the summer to find a job in California.

After the wedding, they settled into an apartment in Los Angeles. Amy found a job teaching at a private school in Beverly Hills. She hated the work. Most of the students were spoiled, she felt. Their parents encouraged irresponsibility, taking them out of class to go skiing in Switzerland or scuba diving in the Caribbean. That was no way to teach children about the things that mattered, Amy thought.

Fortunately, she had other challenges to occupy her. She and Mike had wanted to get started on having a family as soon as possible. She got pregnant a month after the wedding. It was a difficult pregnancy. Amy was sick much of the time, but the months seemed to sail by.

The prospect of having a child in some ways seemed overwhelming. From childhood, Amy had always felt a special sense of closeness with her own mother. Even now, even though Amy was an adult and lived more than 2,000 miles away from Nancy, the two of them still talked on the phone every day. Nancy had a gift for making life seem manageable, for making her daughter's fears melt away.

Amy gave birth to a little girl late in April, 1990. She and Mike named their daughter Sarah. Amy quit teaching so she could stay home with their little girl.

Their daughter's birth gave Mike and Amy a sense of satisfaction that surprised them. The work of taking care of a newborn seemed endless. There were the night feedings, the constant concerns about the baby's health, the awkwardness of doing housework with an infant in arm. None of that seemed to matter, though, when Mike and Amy could sit together and watch their daughter. They decided to have more children, and as soon as possible.

When Sarah was a year and a half old, Amy got pregnant again. She went to the doctor one day while Mike was at work. The doctor told her she was carrying twins. The news rocked her. When she thought about caring for three small children, she began to feel panic. She had to talk to Mike.

It wasn't easy reaching him. He was on a construction site and hated to be called while he was working. He thought it was unprofessional to take personal calls on business time. She tracked him down, though, and told him the news. Twins.

Mike's irritation about being distracted at work disappeared. He told Amy that they could manage this, that they could handle almost anything. They wanted children, enough to make a family like the ones they had grown up in. Now they would have them. This was good news, he said.

Later, they talked about the details of caring for their children. They would need help with a toddler and two infants, they decided. They needed to be closer to their families. That meant moving to either Colorado or Indiana.

Mike talked to his supervisors at Oxford. They found a position for him back in Indianapolis. The Hunts were going home.

In Indianapolis, they bought a new house on the city's west side. The house was about a ten-minute drive from Amy's parents' home. Help with the kids would be close by.

The twins were born on June 29, 1992. Mike and Amy named them Emily and Nicole. Once the twins came home, the Hunt family settled into a routine. As in Los Angeles, Amy stayed home with the children. She planned to teach again someday, but not while her kids were small. When they were ready for school, she would think about going back to the classroom. Maybe she could even find a teaching job at the same school the girls were in.

Fatherhood changed Mike, in ways that surprised and pleased Amy. During their courtship and the early days of their marriage, it always had seemed to her that his career came first. He worked long hours, and never seemed to want to be away from the office for long. Now, though, she noticed that he was going into work later and coming home earlier. He liked to linger with his daughters, playing games with them and teasing them. His family had become the center of his life.

As the girls grew, their personalities began to emerge. Sarah was sensitive, a child with surprising empathy. She could understand another person's pain or discomfort and was always the first of the girls to reach out. Nicole was more aggressive and adventurous, a spirited little girl who liked to be where things were happening.

Emily was more quiet and thoughtful, a shy little girl who ran with small skipping steps. For a child, she moved amazingly gracefully, like a tiny dancer. Her parents watched her and told each other, "She will be a ballerina some day."

On that August Saturday in 1996, Grandparents' Weekend did not begin well at the Hunt home. Early in the afternoon, Amy loaded the girls into the car to drive them to Grandma's. This was the first time the twins were old enough to go on Grandparents' Weekend. The girls were excited.

Mike wasn't. Just as they were loading up the car, he had wandered down to the basement of the house, which was the girls' playroom. They had strewn their toys all over the floor in the morning and just left them there. He marched out to the driveway and told his daughters that they wouldn't be going anywhere until they cleaned up the playroom. He threatened to call Grandma and tell her that the girls wouldn't be coming over.

Sarah, Nicole and Emily bolted out of the car and ran down to the basement. They worked so hard at straightening up that they had the basement clean in minutes. Clearly, they really wanted to go to see Grandma and Grandpa.

When the girls finished their chore, Sarah and Nicole ran up to their father to give him a hug and a kiss goodbye. Emily tried to scoot past. That was typical. Unlike her sisters, she was not a toucher, not a little girl who hungered for hugs and kisses. This was particularly true when she was angry about something—like being told to clean the basement when she really wanted to go see Grandma.

Mike laughed, and said, "Don't you want to say goodbye to me?"

Emily skipped over to her father, put her arms around his neck and kissed him quickly on the cheek. Then she loped over to the car and got in.

When Amy and the girls got to Bud and Nancy's house, Amy lingered for a few minutes to talk with her sister-in-law, David's wife, Leslie. They chatted about what they planned to do while the children were with their grandparents. Amy told her that she and Mike hadn't made any really firm plans. They had a party to go to that night, and they intended to go to church in the morning. After that, they hadn't decided. Maybe they would go to Circle Centre Mall to shop.

By the time Amy left Bud and Nancy's and got back home, it was late afternoon. They decided to go out for a nice dinner together before they went to the party. They went to Zorro's, a Mexican restaurant on the city's northside only a couple of miles from the place they had first met. They indulged themselves by lingering over dinner, then went to the party. They stayed long enough to make their presence known, but were home by a little after eleven. As parents of three children, the possibility of a night of uninterrupted sleep was more tantalizing to them than any party could be.

The next morning, they went to church. Afterward, they decided to head straight to the mall. They wanted to see a movie, something they rarely got to do with the children. They couldn't decide if they should eat lunch before they saw the movie, but determined that they really weren't that hungry. On their way to the theater, they stopped at the food court and bought some French fries to share.

They got to the theater, bought tickets and found their seats. The lights went dim and the previews ran across the screen. They held hands. It was nice to have a little time just to be with each other.

Minutes after the opening credits to the movie—"Courage Under Fire"—finished, the mall's public address system began to crackle, then a voice said, "If Michael and Amy Hunt are anywhere in the mall, they should report to the security desk."

Amy felt herself grow short of breath. She looked over at Mike. One glance told her that he was thinking what she was. This was bad.

They gathered their things up and left their seats. When they got to the end of the row, Amy checked her purse. Her wallet was missing. She felt a huge sense of relief. Maybe that's why they were paging her. Maybe someone in the mall had found her wallet.

No, Mike said. People lost wallets all the time, but he'd never heard a p.a. system used to return a billfold. Most likely she had dropped it under the seat. They walked back to where they had been sitting, ran their hands along the floor and found the wallet.

Amy felt a horrible sense of dread overtake her. It seemed as if all the strength had left her legs and arms, as if they had been pounded into putty.

She and Mike found their way to the public security office. The person at the desk told Mike to call the Boone County Sheriff's office, and handed him a phone.

Mike called and the deputy on the other end of the line asked him if he had a four-year-old daughter who might have been at the Old Indiana amusement park that day. If so, she was hurt and Mike needed to get to Methodist Hospital as quickly as possible.

"I have two four-year-old daughters," Mike said. "Can you tell me which one was hurt?"

The deputy told him to go to Methodist. All his questions would be answered there.

After hanging up, Mike told Amy what the deputy had said. She felt even more frightened. They had to hurry, Mike said.

They started walking to the car. Amy had a hard time keeping up. Her legs felt like they would give out. She had never been so scared, so shaken, in all her life. None of this seemed real. She just wanted to sit down and wait for it to go away.

Come on, Mike kept saying. We have to hurry, he said, pulling her along.

Once they got to the car, Amy began to collect herself. A thought cut through the shock. One of her little girls was hurt. She needed to be with her daughter. The hospital was seventeen blocks from the mall. She told Mike to run red lights to get there. Every time he slowed the car at an intersection to check for traffic, she yelled, "Go, go, go!"

They got to the hospital, and ran to the front desk. They told the woman there who they were. She led them to a waiting room where the rest of the family was gathered.

Amy's sister Kathy ran up to them. She was crying, and looked like she had been crying for quite a while.

Kathy said there had been an accident at the park—a bad accident.

"Mom's gone and Emily might not make it," Kathy said.

Amy couldn't understand what Kathy was saying. What

did Kathy mean by saying Mom was gone, Amy asked. Where did their mother go?

"No," Kathy said gently, "Mom's dead."

Amy felt her legs give way beneath her. She fainted, collapsing on the floor.

Some nurses took Amy to a recovery room. Mike tried to find out what had happened. The family told him as much as they knew. He knew that a train had wrecked, and he learned that much of the family had been on it when it left the tracks. Nancy and Emily had been hurt the worst, but almost everyone on the train had something bruised or broken. All of his daughters had wounds from the wreck.

The nurses told him that he and Amy couldn't see Emily just then, so he went off in search of Sarah and Nicole. He found them. Sarah had suffered a concussion and some lacerations on her face. She had to have stitches. Sarah was not a girl to endure pain stoically. She held onto her father's hand fiercely, tears streaming down her face.

She kept asking, "What about Grandma? Is Grandma all right?"

Mike tried to put off telling her, but Sarah was insistent. She had seen her grandmother lying in a heap at the park and was old enough to know that Nancy's injuries were serious. Mike finally told his daughter that her grandmother had died.

Sarah cried even harder, and then looked up at her father.

"Oh, Daddy, what's Grandpa going to do?" she asked. "He's going to be so lonely."

Mike had to turn his head away to keep from crying himself.

Nicole hadn't been hurt as bad. She had been bruised and banged up. When she saw Mike, she looked at him and shook her head.

"Daddy," she said, "that train started to go crazy, so I jumped off it and ran over to the fence."

Mike smiled in spite of himself. Most likely, he knew, the train wreck had thrown her against the fence, but that was Nicole. She was a little girl who didn't like to admit to being afraid.

Kathy came into the room. She told Mike the doctors had said that he and Amy could see Emily now.

When he got to the emergency room, Amy was already there. After she recovered, she pushed her way into the emergency room, just to let Emily know that her mother was there. The nurses had led Amy away, but not before she had seen her daughter immobilized on an operating table with tubes attached to her.

Now Amy stood with her husband looking at their daughter. The doctors whispered about Emily's injuries. A broken neck. Broken arm. Broken jaw.

As the doctors spoke in hushed tones, Mike prayed. "Please don't let there be anything wrong with this little girl's mind," he asked God. "We can deal with anything else."

The doctors assured him that Emily had not suffered a brain injury.

Mike mouthed a silent thank you and then changed his prayer.

"Please let my little girl live," he begged.

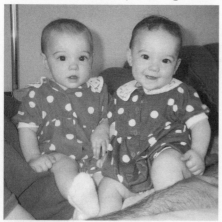

Nikki, (left) and Emily sit on their father's lap during their first spring.

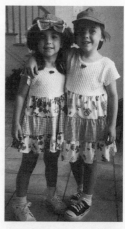

Emily, (left) and Nikki on their fourth birthday, a few weeks before the tragedy.

CHAPTER FOUR

W̲HEN THE TINY TRAIN AT THE O̲LD I̲NDIANA F̲AMILY F̲UN-N-
Water Park jumped the tracks, the resulting tragedy bought the Hunt and Jones families membership into two
surprisingly large yet largely unknown societies of suffering.

The two groups: Americans who have suffered life-alter-
ing or life-ending accidents at amusement parks and Americans who have suffered spinal cord injuries.

Neither group gets the attention it deserves, in part because most Americans prefer to think that all amusement
parks are safe and that spinal cord injuries are very rare.

In thinking that way, most Americans are wrong—perhaps for understandable reasons, but wrong nonetheless.

It's not surprising, for example, that most people want
to believe that all amusement parks are safe. Like Bud Jones,
they think of amusement parks as near-sanctuaries for children, places where innocence will be protected at all costs.
Most people do not like to think that some business people
and some government officials might be careless with
children's lives.

But they are. Between 1987 and 1999, forty-three people
in twenty-three different states died in amusement park accidents. In addition, in *every year* since 1994, at least 7,000 people
per year have been injured in amusement park accidents.

If anything, the trend is upward. In 1994, there were 7,400
amusement park ride injuries in the United States. Five years
later, in 1999, the number had climbed by nearly 2,000 injuries to 9,200—a jump of twenty-four percent.

Two sets of circumstances generally led to accidents. The
first, not surprisingly, was the sheer number of people going

to the parks and taking the rides. In the period from 1987 to 1999, New York led the nation in amusement park deaths with five, and three other big states—California, Florida and Texas—followed closely with four apiece.

The other factor, though, is not necessarily related to size. The parks in states that have strict regulations for rides and thorough inspection practices generally saw fewer accidents and fewer deaths.

A few states—Alabama, Kansas, Missouri, Montana, North Dakota, South Dakota, Utah and Vermont—don't even require inspections. Still others may require inspections, but do not provide sufficient training for the people who are supposed to perform the inspections.

For this reason—and because the numbers of accidents had climbed so dramatically—in May of 2000 the chairwoman of Consumer Product Safety Commission called for the federal government to establish national regulations for amusement parks. Ann Brown, the CPSC chairwoman, said that the lives of America's children were too precious to leave to risk.

The Hunts certainly would have agreed with Brown.

The second society the family joined following the wreck at Old Indiana was that of the Americans who have spinal cord injuries.

Because the idea of paralysis is so disturbing, it is tempting to think that only a handful of people experience it. The facts say otherwise.

Right now, more than 250,000 people in the United States have experienced a spinal cord injury that has left them either as a paraplegic or a quadriplegic. Another 11,000 join their ranks every year. That's another thirty *every day*. Or, another one every forty-five minutes.

Most of these folks are in the prime of life when they get injured. The average age is thirty-one.

When their spines get damaged, they face a daunting set of challenges. The cost of their initial hospitalization, therapy and re-entry into their own homes costs at least $140,000.

Generally, the medical care and therapy they will require over the course of their lifetime will be at least another $400,000. Often, it exceeds a million dollars.

Taken as a whole, spinal cord injuries cost American taxpayers roughly 10 billion dollars annually—not to speak of the additional billions spent on veterans' benefits and disability payments that are never counted. The drain on the economy is even greater. It is estimated that, each year, spinal cord injuries and brain disorders add up to 400 billion dollars in lost productivity and other direct and indirect costs.

The sad thing is that researchers estimate that spending another 300 million to 500 million dollars would produce a cure. That doesn't seem like a high price to pay to help a quarter of a million people walk again.

The human costs for not spending the money are immeasurable.

The typical spinal cord injury victim, for example, is a young male just past the age of thirty.

He is married.

He has children.

Most likely, his injury has left him a quadriplegic—meaning that movement and control in all four of his limbs has been affected.

Chances are, he lives in a wheelchair.

Insurance can cover many of the costs of his hospitalization and his therapy. Sound financial planning may be able to allow him to provide for his family's welfare. But what of the other things in his life—the things that give his life meaning?

What kind of price should be put on a husband's inability to hold his wife?

A father's frustration at not being able to give his child a hug?

Or, for that matter, the shattered dreams of a four-year-old girl who wanted to be ballerina when she grows up?

Spinal cord injuries shatter lives just as surely as they

damage spines. They derail dreams, strain marriages and bankrupt families.

And this tragedy replays itself thirty times every day.

Emily Hunt was one of those tragedies.

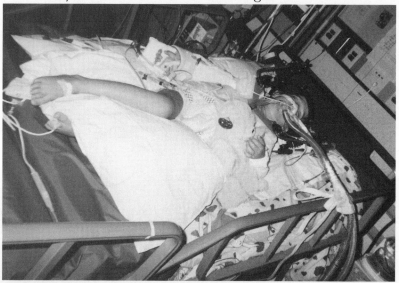

Emily waits at Riley Hospital to have a tracheotomy. Up to that point, Emily still could make her voice heard.

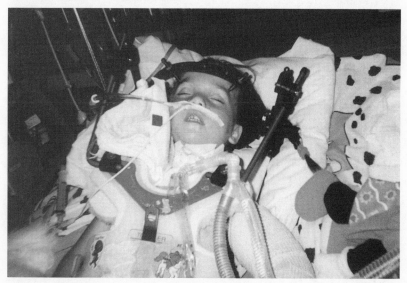

After the tracheotomy, Emily's voice went silent. She could only communicate by blinking.

CHAPTER FIVE

A MY WAS HAUNTED BY SOMETHING ONE OF THE DOCTORS HAD told her about Emily. Oddly, it wasn't about the most significant of Emily's injuries—the fracturing of her spine. Minutes after Mike and Amy arrived at the hospital, the doctors told them how serious Emily's injuries were. It was unlikely, the doctors said, that Emily ever would walk again. The words washed over Amy like a wave, then receded. Like the news of Nancy's death, the thought that Emily would go through life paralyzed was too horrible for Amy to accept at once. She didn't want it to be true.

Speaking matter-of-factly, the doctor described Emily's broken jaw as if he were a stamp collector discussing a rare find. He said that it was unusual for a child as young as Emily break her jaw, much less break it in three places as Emily had. Children's bones were so soft that it was difficult for them to break. For Emily's jaw to be broken the way it was, the impact must have been like a missile hitting a target.

As the doctor talked, Amy could see her four-year-old daughter flying through the air and crumpling against a tree. The thought sickened her.

For a while, Mike stood close to Emily and looked at her. He considered himself a tough-minded man, one who could confront reality without flinching, but he found it hard to look at his daughter while the doctors worked on her. When Emily hit the tree at the park, the impact had opened a huge laceration in the back of her head. The doctors had stapled it shut. She had a tube running into her mouth. The doctors did tests, running an MRI and a CAT scan to determine the extent of Emily's injuries. Whenever they shifted her or tried to work on Emily's broken arm, the little girl grimaced.

Those moments sent jolts through Mike, almost as if he had been hit himself. Seeing staples in the back of her head made him feel weak. He stood there for a while, wondering how something so devastating could have happened. His daughter looked so frail, so wounded. Seeing her in so much pain drained Mike of energy. He just wanted to collapse.

Then he roused himself. Standing around feeling bad about his daughter wasn't helping Emily, wasn't helping Amy, wasn't helping his other daughters, wasn't helping anyone. His family needed him. He had to come through.

Amy, he knew, would stay close to Emily to confer with the doctors and whisper reassurances to the little girl. He needed to check again on Sarah and Nicole, then find a place for his daughters to stay that night. He needed to find out what Emily's medical options were, needed to find out who would give her the best care. He needed to call his parents, tell them what had happened and ask them to come out to help.

As soon as he begin putting together plans, he felt his fatigue fade away. In a funny way, it almost reminded him of his days on the rodeo circuit. The trick, he felt, was finding a way to be comfortable with chaos and staying focused on what really mattered. Back then, he worried about staying on the back of the bull. Now, he needed to stay on top of this crisis. He needed to take care of his family.

The doctors talked to him about Sarah's concussion. She could leave the hospital, but she had to be watched closely. If she started to throw up, she would have to come back. Except for a few bumps and bruises, Nicole was fine, and could leave, too.

Sitting on his lap in the waiting room, Sarah made it clear that she wanted to go home, that she wanted to rest in her own bed. She cried, and asked her father to take her back to the house. Mike could understand why she was so upset. If Nancy hadn't died and Emily's injuries weren't so serious, everyone in the family would be huddled around Sarah at the moment, giving her love and sympathy. Instead, people sat in the waiting room almost like zombies, as if they were afraid to move because they might cause some other dreadful thing to happen.

Mike decided that Sarah deserved to be around family and to have someone smothering her with attention. He talked with his brother-in-law, David Hoalt, who said that Sarah and Nikki could spend the night at their house. Before David could take the girls, though, he had to go up to Thorntown to pick up the family cars that had been left at the amusement park. Mike asked some neighbors who had come to the hospital to help if Sarah could stay with them for a little while. They said yes, and took Sarah with them. Nikki wanted to stay at the hospital.

Mike tried to call his parents in Colorado, but got their answering machine. He didn't leave a message. News like this couldn't be left on a machine.

When David got back from picking up the cars, Mike drove over to pick up Sarah and take her out to the Hoalts' house. He dropped Sarah off, then picked up his cell phone to try his parents again while he drove back to the hospital. He listened to the ring and thought he was going to get the machine again, when his mother picked up.

They had just gotten back home from church, she said. Then she asked how Mike was doing.

Mike took a deep breath. Not great, he said.

Then he told his mother about the wreck at the amusement park. He told her that Nancy was dead. Emily had a spinal injury, he said, and the doctors weren't sure that she would live.

As he spoke, he could hear his mother gasp, then grow silent. Mike told her that he really needed their help. He needed it as soon as possible. He asked if she and his father could come out to Indiana to help him and Amy put their family back together.

His mother said they would be out as soon as they could get packed and find a flight.

After he hung up, while he drove back to hospital, Mike had a few minutes to himself. He began to think about the wreck that had broken his daughter's neck. He thought about how Nancy was dead and Emily had metal screws drilled into her skull. How could a children's ride have caused all that? Someone must have really screwed up, he thought. Someone killed his mother-in-law. Someone broke his daughter's spine.

He felt anger surge in him. He fought the feeling down. Stay in control, he told himself. Don't get thrown, he thought. He took a deep breath. When he exhaled, he realized he had been gripping the steering wheel so hard that his hands hurt.

Sheriff Ern Hudson paced around in the waiting room with the family. He had spent most of the day at the Old Indiana park. He still was wearing his red Boone County Sheriff's Department T-shirt. There were sweat stains in the armpits and down the back. His comb-over hairstyle had been blown askew by the day's breezes.

He wanted to express his condolences to the family and assure them that he and his officers would push their investigation as hard as the law allowed. Even though he and Ken Campbell were a long way from knowing exactly why the train had jumped the tracks, Ern had been a cop long enough to know that the people who ran the park weren't telling him the truth. They claimed that the train basically was in good shape, and that it had been inspected often. The maintenance people at Old Indiana had told him that they inspected the train every day. Even if they didn't, the state was supposed to inspect the rides several times a year. Ern had seen the state's records. He knew that state inspectors supposedly had checked the train on July 23—less than three weeks before the wreck.

That told Ern a lot. He had seen the train, and studied the rusted, broken parts. That kind of wear-and-tear didn't show up in three weeks time. That ride hadn't been thoroughly inspected on July 23. It couldn't have been.

Other parts of the story he had been told didn't ring true, either. One of the maintenance people told him that the train wasn't supposed to go any faster than eight miles per hour. The train might have gone a little bit faster than that, but not much, Ern had been told.

Ern knew better. He had investigated a lot of automobile wrecks. He had seen enough accident victims to know what a wreck at eight miles an hour did to a human being. Wrecks at low speeds didn't leave bodies mangled the way Nancy Jones' had been. Wrecks at ten miles an hour didn't crumple little girls like rag dolls.

When he was out at the park, Ern's first duty had been to see that the victims were taken care of. He focused on their injuries, not on their names or identities. He hadn't known right away that seven of the eight people hurt in the wreck belonged to the same family.

Now he did. He shook his head. This was a family who needed help. The grandmother had been killed. The grandfather had had his leg broken. One granddaughter had a broken neck. Another had a concussion. A great aunt had a broken arm. Three other kids had severe bruises. All in one family. All because of a train no taller than a child's bicycle.

His daughter Kathy told Bud that someone wanted to talk to him.

"Who?" Bud asked. A big guy wearing a red T-shirt, Kathy said. She thought he was from the park.

For most of the afternoon and evening, Bud had been

in a haze. The doctors had given him a powerful painkiller. He had faded in and out of consciousness. A lot of people had come by to express their condolences and see how he was doing. Because of the medication, the string of visits confused Bud. Time seemed to be folding up on him.

This visitor, though, Bud wanted to see. In those moments when his head was clear, Bud couldn't stop thinking of how Nancy had looked after she hit the tree. He imagined how scared she must have been in the instant when she was flying through the air. He remembered how cold her leg had been when he touched her.

Bud had never felt rage in his life, but he felt it now. It chased away some of his stupor. He wanted to tell this visitor from the park what Old Indiana's incompetence had cost Bud. Had cost the Jones family.

The visitor came into the room. He was big, a heavy guy who seemed to lurch when he walked.

Before Bud had a chance to say a word, the man introduced himself. "I'm Ern Hudson, sheriff of Boone County. We're gonna be investigating the accident," he said.

Bud didn't say anything. He couldn't. This seemed too strange. He had expected someone from the park, and instead he had this big, clumsy-looking sheriff standing beside him. The drugs slowed Bud's thinking down. He needed a moment to adjust.

The sheriff kept talking. He said that he was sorry that all this had happened to Bud's family. He mentioned Nancy, and said that her death was a horrible loss. He spoke slowly and with a heavy drawl.

The sheriff seemed sincere, but he was not the sort of man who inspired much confidence. Bud listened to the man talk, and winced when the sheriff swore or used "ain't" instead of "isn't." The sheriff seemed rough, even crude.

Bud felt himself grow tired again. Once he realized that he wouldn't be able to tell someone from Old Indiana about the damage the park had done to his family, his energy seemed to drift away. He wanted to be angry; instead, he just felt weary and alone. He wanted the man in the red shirt to go away so he could rest quietly.

Then the sheriff said something that made Bud pay attention. In that slow drawl, the big man said, "Bud, listen carefully. You need to get yourself a lawyer. You need to secure that site. This shouldn't have happened, and you need to take care of your family."

Bud shifted his head and made a weak motion with his hand. The sheriff read the signal and realized Bud wanted to say something. Maybe the big man understood more than he let on.

Bud was too weak to speak in much more than a whisper. The words came out in a rasp.

"Don't let this happen to anyone else's family," Bud said.

The sheriff nodded and promised to do his best.

As midnight approached, Mike and Amy settled in for a long wait. The evening had been a busy one.

Just as he had returned to the hospital, Mike had gotten a call from his brother-in-law. Sarah had started throwing up—one of the warning signs the doctors had talked about. Mike ran out to get her.

On the way, his pickup started jerking and sputtering. He looked at the dashboard. The needle on the gas gauge hovered on "E." With everything else going on, he hadn't even noticed.

There was a gas station up ahead. He threw the car into neutral and let it drift up to the pump. Trouble had been averted, just barely. He hoped his luck would hold.

After he picked up Sarah, he got word that his parents would be arriving around 11 pm. That made things easier. The girls could stay in their home with their grandmother and grandfather. As scared and shaken up as the girls were, it would help to have family around.

The doctors released Sarah again. She went home with Mike's parents, the folks she called Papa Bob and Grandma Kay.

Mike joined Amy. Now that their other daughters were being taken care of, they both wanted to be close to their little girl. They sat, holding hands, and waited.

The waiting was difficult. The doctors weren't encouraging. They told Mike and Amy that Emily might not live. Even if she did, it wasn't likely that she would walk again. If Emily didn't show some signs of movement in the next few days, it most likely would mean that her paralysis was permanent.

Amy kept trying to wish her daughter out of the hospital and back onto her feet. Amy wanted to see Emily skipping along like a ballerina again. Even more, Amy wanted reassurance, some guarantee, that her daughter would live. Amy couldn't imagine her little girl dead. But Amy had never imagined that her mother would die this soon, and yet Nancy was dead. Amy felt weak and so vulnerable that it almost hurt to breathe. Fear seemed to squeeze her. It seemed to Amy that she had taken so much for granted. She had assumed that Emily would grow up healthy—assumed that Nancy would be just a few miles and a phone conversation away.

She squeezed her husband's hand.

Mike spent the time thinking about his family's needs. The doctors' news made him realize that those needs were larger than he could have thought. Emily was going to need extensive care. It would be expensive. Mike knew his health insurance policy had a million-dollar cap. From what the doctors were saying, Emily's care could cost that much in just the next few weeks. How would he take care of her after that? He needed to talk to a lawyer.

Amy looked down at her watch, and noticed something strange. It had quit working. The hands were frozen at ten minutes to noon, the time the train had left the tracks. The time when her mother died, when Emily hit the tree.

The coincidence gave Amy a chill. She showed the watch to Mike. He shook his head in wonder, and gripped his wife's hand a little more tightly.

CHAPTER SIX

During all her hours at the hospital, Amy knew that there was at least one essential thing she had left undone. She had not said goodbye to her mother. She wanted to see her mother's body before the casket was closed.

Bud resisted the idea. He had been at the wreck and knew what kind of damage had been done to Nancy. He tried to talk Amy out of looking at her mother's body. He told his daughter that she should remember her mother the way Nancy had been in life, not the way Nancy's body looked now. The morticians at Conkle's Funeral Home had done their best to make Nancy look the way she did before the wreck, but it was a difficult task. She had been thrown headfirst into a tree at a high speed, and her features had been severely distorted by the impact.

Amy insisted.

When Amy came to the funeral home, she went straight to the casket. She had not left the hospital since the accident. She planned to be away from Emily for a few minutes at the calling and then for the funeral the next day, a Friday. She had not had much time to think about her mother's death. Her daughter's care consumed all of Amy's energy and concentration.

Amy looked down at her mother's body. The body in the casket looked nothing like the woman who had raised Amy and had taught her almost everything she knew about being a wife and a mother. Amy snapped into a rage.

"That's not my mother! That's not my mother!" Amy screamed.

She broke into tears, long, wailing sobs. Bud hobbled over to her on his broken leg and tried to comfort his youngest daughter. Amy kept yelling that it wasn't her mother in the casket. It couldn't be.

As her father held her, Amy began to gasp out words, half-articulated snatches of grief and explanation. She wailed that she missed her mother. That she needed Nancy now more than she ever had. That she was furious with the people who had been careless enough to let her mother die and break her child's spine.

The anger spilled out of her, as if it had overrun a vessel. Bud listened to Amy, and ached.

After her sobbing ended, Amy told her father that this wasn't the way she wanted to remember her mother, stretched out like a wax figure in a museum. Nancy wouldn't want to have her friends see her that way either.

It was better, Amy said, to remember Nancy alive, in one of her color-coordinated outfits playing with her children and grandchildren.

Bud hugged his daughter. They asked the people at the funeral home to close the casket.

The hours leading up to Nancy's funeral filled Bud with an overwhelming sense of numbness. In every other time of crisis in his life, he always had been able to turn to his wife. He had always been able to count on Nancy.

Bud felt that a lot had gone right in his life, but nothing had gone more right than marrying Nancy. They had been together since the eighth grade. Back then, he had been a boy with an open, wholesome face and cheeks like the little Dutch boy on the paint cans. Nancy had dark hair and a fast smile. They had come together because of a shared need. They both had been sensitive children in homes that had known some measure of unhappiness. Bud's father was a drinker. Watching his father drink away his family's money and security left

Bud with a lifelong abhorrence of excess and irresponsibility. Nancy's parents were decent people who loved her, but they could be distant and uncommunicative. That could make things uncomfortable for a young woman as open and friendly as she was. Nancy regarded love the same way she regarded air, as something fundamental to life. She could no more hold back her concern and affection than she could stop her heart from pounding.

While they were both in junior high, Nancy quickly fell into the habit of making Bud's house her second home, maybe even her real home. That was all right with Bud. He knew from the beginning that this was the girl for him, the one who would make the pieces of his life fit together. She was pretty, with her big round eyes and a figure of compacted roundness. She was so kind and so capable that she made him feel that nothing could go truly wrong in his life. They could deal with anything.

Bud and Nancy were one of those couples everyone expected to do well. They were friendly, well-liked and obviously in love. After high school, they opted not to go to college, in large part because they wanted to get married—to get on with the business of starting their life together and building a family.

The early years of their marriage had not been without hardship. Bud found work at a company that manufactures parts for household appliances and began a steady climb up the corporate ladder. Nancy stayed home to take care of the children. Money was tight. As young marrieds, their closest friends were Bud's sister Polly and her husband Bob. A big night out involved having one couple visit the other for an evening of card playing. The couple doing the visiting brought their own soda pop and potato chips, because neither family could afford to entertain in even modest style.

Even though the money wasn't plentiful, Bud figured that he and Nancy had been fortunate in other ways. Before they knew it, they had three healthy children, Kathy, David and

Amy. As parents, he and Nancy figured that the most important lessons they could teach their kids were the old-fashioned
ones. They raised their children to be honest, to work hard
and to honor their commitments.

Most of all, Bud and Nancy drilled home the importance
of family. Family was the one thing a person should be able to
count on in both good times and bad. Every evening, the
children were expected home for dinner. That was family time.
Over supper, the kids would talk about school, about their
friends, about their plans for the weekend. If any member of
the family, parent or child, had a problem, the dinner table
was the place where it got thrashed out. The dinner hour itself was flexible; supper could take anywhere from twenty
minutes to four hours, depending upon the subjects up for
discussion. Attendance, though, was mandatory. No one in the
Jones family missed dinner without a good excuse.

Before the accident, Bud figured he and Nancy had done
their job as parents pretty well. Now that he and his wife were
both in their mid-fifties, all their children were grown and in
happy, stable marriages themselves. He had a bunch of grandchildren who loved to come to Grandpa and Grandma's
house.

Right up until the moment the train jumped the tracks
at the amusement park, he had felt that he was an extremely
fortunate man.

And now he was getting ready to go bury his wife.

It seemed to Amy as if everyone in Indianapolis came to
the funeral home that day. Family members, friends, acquain-
tances, even people she barely knew came by to tell her how
sorry they were. The funeral home wasn't far from the Indianapolis Motor Speedway, where the Indianapolis 500 took
place every May. Sometimes, when drivers died at the track,
the services were held at Conkle's. The funeral director was
accustomed to large crowds, he told Amy. Even so, he said he

had never seen one like this.

That seemed odd to Amy, too. The train wreck had made her family's life a public story. The first night at the hospital she had looked out the window and seen the bright lights the television cameras on the grass. She told Mike that there must be some big story going on at the hospital. Mike shook his head and told her, "We're the story. We're the reason they're here."

Amy didn't particularly like that. She enjoyed being a private person, never wanted to be the center of attention. Amy liked quiet things, and took comfort in life's ordinary pleasures, like talking to her mother on the phone every day. Or watching Emily run with those graceful, skipping strides.

Now that was gone, and she felt as if her family's pain was on display. Total strangers talked about Nancy and Emily as if they knew her mother and daughter. There was a kindness, a concern, to their talk, but occasionally their polite chatter cut Amy like tiny nicks from a knife.

People came up to her and said that her mother had been prepared to die, that Nancy had lived fully. Those people meant well. They were trying to comfort her, Amy knew. But their words stoked her anger.

Her mother hadn't been ready to die. Amy knew that. Nancy wanted to live. Nancy wanted to see her "babies"—her grandchildren—as often as she could. She wanted to have more grandparents' weekends. Wanted to see grandchildren grow up and go to college. Wanted to grow old with Amy's father, and enjoy the comfortable lifestyle they had devoted decades to building.

Amy wasn't ready for her mother to die, either. Motherhood was the biggest challenge of Amy's life, and she depended on Nancy for advice and support. Emily was in the hospital. The doctors couldn't even assure Amy and Mike that their daughter would live, much less be healthy again.

Amy needed her mother's counsel more than ever, but Nancy was gone. Gone.

The morning of the funeral, David Jones came by his parents' house to pick up Bud. On his way to the front door, David saw a dove flying overhead.

Bud found it hard to get around. His broken leg made it impossible for him to drive and difficult for him to walk. It seemed that all he could do was sit and think about his wife.

The funny thing was, he and Nancy had talked about death. It was something parents had to do, particularly once they started to get a little older. In some ways, talking about it seemed almost comforting, as if by discussing death they could keep it bay, push it far into the future. He and Nancy agreed that, whichever one of them died first, they each would want the other to go on, to try to find a way to live and be happy again.

It sounded good at the time. Those talks, though, always dealt with another time, when they both would be in their late seventies or early eighties. Finding a way to be happy meant struggling to make life's last days pleasant. Bud was fifty-six. He still had a lot of years to live. He never thought he would have to live them alone. In all their time together, he had never imagined being without Nancy. She seemed as essential to living as his lungs or his heart.

His thoughts never left her. He could not think for long about her or their life together without weeping.

The minister, Dean Dickinson of Chapel Rock Christian Church, knew Nancy. He had been her pastor.

He described her as a woman who loved her family and her friends and took joy in them. He talked of the pleasure she took from being with her grandchildren—how she found special times to be with each of them. He said she had been at peace at the time of her death because she never had turned away a person in need.

The words jolted David. As the oldest son, he always had been a striver, a man focused on his career. Bud put a lot of pressure on him to perform when he was young, and David had struggled to meet his father's expectations. When David grew to manhood, the expectations became his own. It seemed there always was something for him to do at the office, some other work commitment he had to meet.

At family gatherings, he always was the last to arrive and the first to leave. He always figured there would be time to catch up, later. Now, though, his mother was dead. Later was gone.

The violinist played *Lara's Theme*, from *Doctor Zhivago*. It was Nancy's favorite. Whenever the family got together at the Chanteclair Restaurant for their holiday dinner, Nancy always requested the song.

As the violinist played, Bud, Amy, David and Kathy put their arms around each other and sobbed. Little Sarah, Mike and Amy's oldest daughter, sat by her father. Everyone in the family wondered if she was old enough to understand what was going on.

Sarah cried and cried and cried. She understood.

When David took Bud back home, he saw a dove again. He wondered if it was a symbol of his mother's spirit.

The family stayed at Bud's house for a long time that night. David and Kathy were worried about Bud, and they didn't want him to feel that he was alone in his grief. They stayed close to their father, talking about Nancy well into the night.

Eventually, though, they had to go home.

When they did, Bud tried to go to bed. It was no use. He thought about the funeral, about the way he and the family had tried to say goodbye to Nancy earlier in the day. He remembered the way Nancy looked beside the tree, like a rag doll someone had thrown away without a second thought.

He thought about his wife, and found that he could not stop crying.

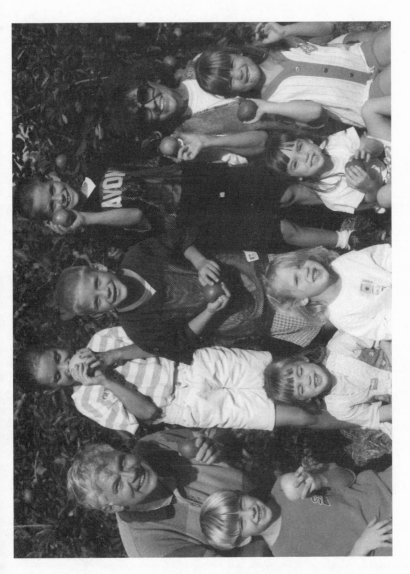

Bud and Nancy with their grandchildren on a previous grandparents' weekend to an apple orchard. (Bk-L) Bud Jones, Kaitlyn Hoalt, Zach Hoalt, Josh Hoalt, Nancy Jones; (Fr-L) Drew Jones, Nikki Hunt, Ellie Jones, Emily Hunt, Sarah Hunt

CHAPTER SEVEN

SOME PARTS OF POLICE WORK ERN HUDSON NEVER QUITE GOT used to. The worst part of the job always had been the notification calls. Too many times, Ern had made the walk up to some stranger's door, knocked, and then delivered the quiet words telling someone that a child, mother, brother or spouse had been killed in an accident or a crime. His words often blew people's lives apart. All that was left after one of those visits was grief.

At one time, Ern had thought that experience would make that part of the job easier. He thought years of working as police officer would make him more callous, less sensitive to the suffering of others. He had started as a state trooper when he was twenty-one, one of the youngest in Indiana. Back then, he figured that time would toughen him, harden him to his task as a bearer of bad news.

It hadn't turned out that way. At forty-six, after twenty-five years of work as a cop, he found it more difficult than ever to tell people that they had lost a loved one. Growing older had taught him something about the fragility of life, and about the ways that human beings have to count on one another. He couldn't help but feel that every death, every loss, touched him in some way.

The night of the Old Indiana wreck, when Ern stopped at the hospital, he and Ken Campbell tried to talk to Amy Hunt. The poor woman was so distraught that she couldn't speak. Her mother was dead, and all three of her children had been injured, one of them so seriously that it seemed she might die. It all seemed to overwhelm Amy. When Ken and Ern tried to express their condolences, her mouth began to move almost spastically, as if she were trying to form words but couldn't, but no sounds came out.

Later, Ern and Ken talked about that moment. Like Bud Jones, they both were traditional men who believed in caring for their families at all costs. Like Bud, they both married their high school sweethearts and began their families when they were young.

Both Ern and Ken had taken their children to Old Indiana. It wasn't hard for either man to put himself in Bud Jones' place. Each man thought, *that could have been me. That could have been my family.*

Ern, in particular, could imagine what it was like. His daughters weren't that much younger than Amy Hunt. Thinking of one of them in that kind of anguish cut through him like a saw.

Ern and Ken pledged that they were going to find out what ~~the hell~~ went wrong out at Old Indiana.

When Ken got his hands on the little train's maintenance log, he found that the records had been altered. Someone had used white-out to erase old entries and write in new ones. In places, the ink and the white liquid were so fresh that they were gooey to the touch.

He tried to question maintenance people about the accident, but the park's attorney, Kent Frandsen, demanded that Ken stop asking questions. The lawyer said that a story in a local newspaper had cast the park in a bad light. Ken wondered how a wreck that killed a grandmother and left a four-year-old girl hovering near death could be put in a good light.

After the attorney ended the interview, a representative from the state fire marshal's office showed up to serve notice that the park was being shut down while the investigation took place. The park's managers were furious.

When Ken started to drive out the park's gate, the park's president, Don Taylor, flagged him down. Ken stopped and rolled down his car window.

Taylor tore into him. Taylor said that the way the sheriff's department was conducting the investigation was outrageous. He said that he had worked in the amusement business all over the country. Accidents happened but business had to go on, he shouted. In all his years in the amusement park business, Taylor said, he had never seen an accident investigated this way.

Ken smiled at the amusement park president and wished him a good day. Then he drove away thinking that, without really meaning to, Taylor had paid the sheriff's department quite a compliment.

The park's attorney decided to turn up the heat on the sheriff's department. Frandsen told every reporter who would listen to him that Ern Hudson was conducting a vendetta, that he was trying to drive a local business under.

Publicly, Ern laughed about it. If someone asked him about Fransden's comments, he said he didn't even know what "vendetta" meant, much less know how to conduct one.

In private, though, Ern experienced a different reaction. He knew what Fransden and the park's owners were trying to do. Lebanon was a small town where jobs, once lost, were not easily replaced. By attacking him as anti-business, the park's owners were trying to force the city fathers to pull Ern's leash and make him stop nosing around Old Indiana. They wanted to put enough pressure on Ern to make him stop.

Other people had tried doing that to Ern in the past, and it always made him angry.

When he was twenty-eight, with a wife and young children at home, Ern had decided that being a state trooper required him to spend too much time on the road. He wanted to stay closer to his family and put down roots in the community. He decided to run for Boone County Sheriff.

There was a problem, though. The Indiana State Police had a rule that troopers couldn't run for political office. Ern thought that was ridiculous. He didn't believe that he ought to have to give up his rights as a citizen just because he wore a trooper's uniform. He tried to tell his supervisors in the state police that, tried to get them to see reason.

They couldn't. In fact, they took a hard line with Ern and threatened to discipline him, even break him. That didn't sit well with Ern, who figured he had every right to run for public office if he wanted to. Ern got mad, and decided to fight.

He got a lawyer and sued the state of Indiana. He won. Then he ran for sheriff and won again. By sticking to his guns, Ern got exactly what he wanted—a chance to continue doing police work while staying closer to his home.

But it wasn't exactly the way he wanted it. All in all, he would have preferred to do everything the easy way and find some solution that allowed everyone to get along. But, if other folks wanted to play rough, that was fine with Ern, too. He was big enough to handle the rough stuff.

Now, nearly twenty years later, someone else was trying to squeeze Ern, trying to keep from doing something he thought was right. Ern didn't like it. Not one bit.

The physical evidence Ern and Ken found chilled them.

The little train was supposed to have thirty-two derailing clamps. The clamps were designed to keep the train on the track and upright. On the day of the wreck, only three of those clamps were in place.

Most of the brakes also were gone. One long section of the track had been welded amateurishly in a vain attempt to keep the train from jumping the tracks. And, right up next to the engine was an open gas container with fuel sloshing around in it.

The more they looked at it, the more Ern and Ken began to think that the accident could have been far, far worse. If the train had tipped a few seconds later, those riding it would have been thrown into a thicker stand of trees. More of the riders would have sustained injuries as severe as Nancy's and Emily's.

Worse still, if the engine had tipped completely and the gasoline from the open container had spilled out so a spark could reach it, there would have been an explosion and a fire. Those sitting closest to the front of the train—almost all of them children—would have been burned severely, and perhaps even killed.

The train, Ern decided, had been a disaster in waiting for months. If it hadn't killed Nancy Jones, it would have killed someone else. It appalled him that the Old Indiana's owners worried so little about the people who came to the park. People like Bud Jones' wife and grandchildren, like Ern's own family.

Ern thought Old Indiana's negligence was criminal, and he wanted to press charges.

Pressing charges wasn't as easy as it looked.

Ern's task was complicated tremendously by one fact. Less than three weeks before the wreck, state inspectors had certified the train as safe. Ern knew from the rust on the ride's derailers and other moving parts that the train's disintegration had been going on for a lot longer than a few days. That ride probably hadn't been safe for more than a year, and maybe even longer than that. He couldn't figure out why any state inspector would give that ride a passing grade.

As he and Ken talked to people at the park, he discovered that the state inspectors knew very little about the rides they were supposed to check. At best, they gave Old Indiana only a cursory examination before they moved on to the next site.

The man who had checked out the train on July 23, nineteen days before the accident, hadn't known how the ride operated. He hadn't looked at the derailers, examined the brakes or even asked park officials to operate the train. In short, his inspection had been worthless.

To everyone but Old Indiana, that is. As long as the park's owners could claim that their ride had met the state's safety standards as recently as three weeks before the wreck, Ern couldn't make a criminal case against them. They could shift the responsibility onto the state, which had immunity from this kind of prosecution.

The only chance that Ern had was to try to prove that the park's owners had conspired to hide the train's true condition from the state's inspectors. If he could do that, he could get around the barrier to prosecution the state's lax inspection presented.

To prove a conspiracy, he had to demonstrate that park officials consistently had falsified records and ordered employees to operate the train regardless of its condition. Ern had a start on making that case. The altered maintenance log gave him one piece of evidence, but he needed something more. That was the testimony of park employees.

Jamie Marquess had told Ern that he frequently had been ordered to run the train even after park officials knew it wasn't safe to operate. Marquess also told the sheriff that maintenance people were pressured to keep the ride going regardless of how many parts were missing.

Ern felt that Marquess was telling him the truth, but, by itself, Marquess's testimony wouldn't be enough to make a persuasive case. Ern needed someone else—someone who would support what Marquess was saying and make ordinary people see how careless the park's owners had been with human lives.

Hard as he tried, Ern couldn't find any other park employee who would go on the record. Most of the people he talked to were terrified that they would lose their jobs and that no other place would hire them if they testified against their employers.

Within a few weeks, Ern discovered that his chances of making a criminal case had vanished.

In the days following the wreck, Ern talked often with Bud.

The two men developed a comfortable relationship. In many ways, they were quite different. One was a slim, soft-spoken businessman. The other was a career cop with a voice that rarely required a megaphone.

But both Ern and Bud felt that men should be responsible for their actions. The fact that Old Indiana seemed to be on the verge of ducking any responsibility for killing Bud's wife—and that the state had helped the park in evading its responsibility—galled both men.

The better he got to know Bud, the more the law officer came to understand the pain the other man was living with. Ern could imagine what it would be like to lose his wife or to see his children hurt. He had delivered bad news hundreds of times, but this time it seemed particularly close, because it had hit a family an awful lot like his.

Ern told Bud that a civil suit probably would be his best bet. Beyond that, Bud and his family might try to get the state to assume some responsibility for the harm that had been done to them. There wasn't any hope for a criminal case. Much as he wanted to, Ern couldn't help Bud.

It hurt Ern quite a bit to say that.

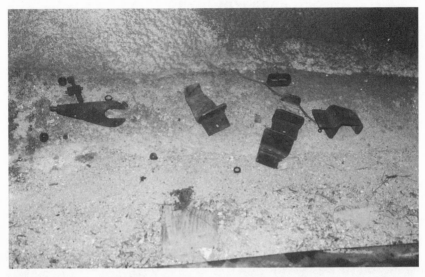

Parts from the train were all strewn along the track. Boone County Sheriff investigators believed the parts had been there a long time.

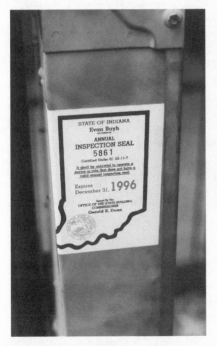

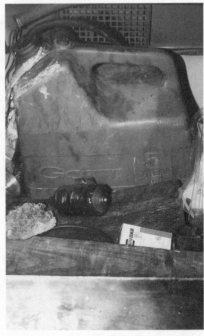

The state's seal of approval that the ride was safe.

An inside view of the train's engine compartment. Note the makeshift gas tank and the uninstalled brake part (NAPA ECHLIN box).

CHAPTER EIGHT

THE DAY AFTER THE WRECK, MIKE AND AMY FOUND THEY HAD a decision to make. The doctors at Methodist kept telling them that Emily was hurt bad, that she might not live, and that even if she did live she would need surgery. The doctors said they had found a small laceration near Emily's spine, and that her spinal cord was dangerously swollen. The doctors wanted to operate.

For a time, Mike and Amy didn't know what to think. The shock of the wreck had yet to wear off. In times of trouble, Amy always had been able to turn to her mother for advice, but Nancy was dead. Amy wanted to be strong, strong enough to care for her children and help her husband, but she had trouble thinking everything through. Part of her wanted to believe that soon all of the turmoil of the past hours would vanish, that the clock would turn itself back to Sunday morning and that she would find her mother and her daughter standing hand-in-hand. The only peace Amy could find came from staying close to Emily, from feeling that she was so close to her little girl that Emily would know that her mother was nearby. Amy could not bear to leave Emily for long. The thought that Emily might feel as alone as Amy felt without Nancy set a snaky kind of fear loose in Amy.

Mike felt the fear, too, but he struggled to beat it down. In those first few hours after the wreck, after he and Amy had rushed to the hospital, he had felt a sense of panic. Now, though, he fought the panic with a kind of cold rationality. His family needed him. His daughter needed him. Making good decisions now was important. If he didn't think things through carefully, his daughter could die or have her life ruined. His family could be ruined.

When he looked at it that way, Mike felt a strange kind of peace come over. In a singular way, that sense of peace resembled the way he felt when he rode bulls in the rodeo. There was chaos and danger all around him, but he felt that all he needed to do was keep his focus and everything would work out.

He started asking the doctors questions about the surgery they wanted to do. Were they the best surgeons for the job? Was there someone who had more experience and a better reputation? Was Emily's age a factor? Wasn't it dangerous to operate on a child so young?

Some of the doctors' answers didn't satisfy Mike, so he began to look for other options. He approached it the way he would approach a business deal. He checked out this possibility and that one, discarding some choices almost as soon they presented themselves and pondering the ones that seemed to give Emily the best chance.

Riley Children's Hospital seemed to offer Emily her best opportunity. The staff there was accustomed to working with small children, and the hospital had one of the best spinal injury surgeons in the country on its staff.

Mike talked with Amy, and they made the decision to move Emily to Riley. Their decision made the doctors at Methodist angry. The doctors told them that they were perfectly competent to give Emily good care. Mike didn't doubt that. Good care, though, wasn't good enough for his little girl. He felt that, even if Emily had only a one-in-a-million chance of walking again, as her father he wanted to make certain that that one chance was the best chance available.

The doctors at Methodist told Mike and Amy that there was a chance Emily wouldn't live through the two-mile ambulance ride to Riley. Emily had been put on a respirator. The air tubes running up into her nose were the only things that kept her breathing. If they got jostled or loosened during the trip, or if Emily stopped breathing for some other reason, she could die. It was foolish, the doctors said, for the Hunts to take such a chance.

Their warnings set Mike and Amy to trembling. Just the day before, a two-mile car ride was an afterthought, a last-minute drive to the grocery store. Now, it could mean life or death for their little girl.

Mike and Amy decided to take the chance. They told the doctors they wanted to move Emily to Riley.

When the time came for Emily to be moved, Mike and Amy held hands, prayed and gave each other hugs. The short ride over seemed unending. Just two days earlier, Mike and Amy had felt like people protected by fate. Now, it was hard for them to believe that the worst thing that could happen wouldn't happen. Every bump seemed ominous. Every jolt made them quiver.

Emily made it through, though, and both Mike and Amy began to feel something they almost had lost—hope. It showed up like an old friend, and immediately began to make Mike and Amy feel a little more comfortable.

Emily's primary care doctor at Riley was Thomas Luerssen, a tall, gray-haired man with a soft voice. Luerssen was the kind of man who radiated calm. He spoke slowly and thoughtfully, spending words as if they were precious coins. His quiet competence inspired confidence.

Luerssen told Mike and Amy that spinal cord surgery for Emily would be a foolish risk. Emily was too young, and had too much growing yet to do. It made more sense to wait.

Then, still speaking quietly, Luerssen told Mike and Amy how serious Emily's injuries were. Emily had broken her arm and her jaw. Those injuries would heal, Luerssen said.

More serious was the injury to Emily's spine. She had a C-7 spinal cord injury—not as bad as the worst spinal cord injuries, but bad enough. Most likely, the doctor said, Emily never would walk again. The impact of being thrown against a tree at nearly forty miles per hour had left Emily's spinal cord swollen and inflamed. The swelling and the inflammation made it impossible for Emily's brain to send signals to her limbs and the rest of her body.

Still talking in his low, soft voice, Luerssen told Amy and Mike that their little girl would need a lot of care. The first challenge, the doctor said, would be to immobilize her and use drugs to try to reduce the swelling of the spinal cord. Because Emily couldn't breathe on her own, she would have to have a tracheotomy and then use a ventilator, which was more reliable than a respirator and would make her breathing more steady. If all went well, Mike and Amy were told, Emily wouldn't need to use the ventilator for long.

Perhaps, the doctor said in his still soft voice, Emily would regain control of her body once the swelling of her spine diminished. The chances were slim, he said, very slim. If her spine had not suffered permanent damage, they should know within a few days, he said.

Mike and Amy held hands, closed their eyes and hoped.

The next day Emily underwent surgery. The Riley doctors wanted to immobilize her. A head brace was the best way to do that.

The brace itself was a gruesome thing. It surrounded the skull and shoulders to hold the spine still and stable. That was the easy part. The difficult part involved the procedure that held the brace in place. In order to keep the thing from slipping, screws had to be drilled into the patient's skull, anchoring the metal brace to the head.

The thought of screws being drilled into his daughter's head made Mike feel weak and queasy, but he knew there was no other option. He wanted her to live, and to have the best chance possible at leading a satisfying life. The head brace represented that chance.

The doctors also performed the tracheotomy and put Emily on a ventilator.

In the days after the operation, Amy and Mike took turns at Emily's bed side, listening to the mechanical wheezing of the ventilator inflating and deflating their daughter's lungs and knowing that it was the only thing that kept their child breathing. The ventilator may have been the device that kept their little girl alive, but its workings—the machine-like rush and push of air it generated—served as a constant reminder of just how tenuous Emily's grasp on life was.

Emily could not speak. Her jaw had been wired shut so the break in it could heal. She took food through a tube. She passed the long hours in the hospital room in silence.

Not long before, Mike and Amy had thought their daughter's voice was one of the sweetest sounds in the world. Now, it was almost a blessing not to hear it.

Emily was in pain most of the time. She was too small and too young to take really potent painkillers, so she had to endure the pain she was feeling. She had to live with the fear, too.

Many hours, Mike and Amy watched and whispered encouragement while their little girl cried. The tears streamed down her face. She didn't make a sound, because she couldn't.

The days, weeks and months following the wreck disappeared in a blur. Mike and Amy found that their lives fell into an exhausting rotation.

One parent was always at Riley with Emily while the other tried to spend enough time at home to keep both the family and the house running. The only time they weren't at home or the hospital was the day of Nancy's funeral. Amy took two hours to attend her mother's service, then hurried back to her daughter's side.

Amy started keeping a journal. She began it almost as a kind of therapy, a means of figuring out what had happened to her and her family. She wrote in it almost religiously, scribbling down both her hopes and her fears. She felt that she had to be strong and stable for her daughters—that she had to take both good news and bad news in stride for their sake.

In her journal, though, she could cast aside stoicism. She wrote about the hope she felt when a doctor or a nurse tapped Emily's leg and it jumped. Amy knew, of course, that the response was a reflex and meant nothing. But it was hard—almost impossible, in fact—not to wish for it to be something more. A miracle, maybe. The beginning of her daughter's recovery to complete health.

Amy wrote about her deepest hopes. She wrote about how much she wanted to see her daughter walk again and about the light, skipping way Emily ran. She wrote about her little girl's dream to grow up and be a dancer.

Amy also wrote about her anger and her loneliness. Her mother's absence seemed like a living, snarling thing, a dangerous creature that could consume her. Well-meaning people had told Amy that Nancy had made her peace and therefore had been prepared to leave the world, but Amy knew better. She knew that her mother had not been ready to die. Amy knew that Nancy had wanted to grow old with Bud and to see all of her grandchildren grow to adulthood.

In her journal, Amy gave vent to her anger about her mother's death. Amy was not a woman who swore easily or often, but swearing seemed to be the only way to release her anger. She wrote in her journal that she was "pissed" that her mother was dead—"pissed" at Old Indiana, "pissed" at the inspectors who said the ride was okay, "pissed" at everyone who had brought this pain and loss to her family.

Amy underlined the word "pissed" three times.

Mike spent more time at home than Amy did.

He saw the way the wreck had affected the other two girls. They both had a hard time accepting the fact that that one moment when the train jumped the tracks had changed their lives forever.

Sarah was old enough to understand that her grandmother was dead, and that death was permanent. Nikki, though, could not grasp that. Occasionally, she would ask, almost timidly, about Nancy. Mike would explain that Nancy had gone to heaven, and Nikki would nod her head as if she understood. But she didn't.

Both girls asked about their sister all the time.

"How's Emily doing?" they asked.

Then, more plaintively, they asked, "When's Emily coming home? Shouldn't Emily be coming home?"

Mike tried to talk to them quietly and in a comforting way about Emily.

He tried to tell them that their sister had been hurt bad, but that she was working really hard at getting better. He tried to tell his little girls that their sister would be home soon, that their family would be complete again before long. He tried to give them the things a father should give his children, the sense that there was someone looking out for them and taking care of them.

But he knew they wanted something else, something more. They wanted to feel that, eventually, things would go back to the way they were before the wreck.

That was the one thing he couldn't give them.

For the longest time in the hospital, Emily did not ask about her grandmother. She could signal or indicate when she wanted to ask a question, and she often did.

She asked about her sisters, about her grandfather and about her cousins. She knew they were all right, because she had seen them at the hospital, so the questions were safe ones for her to ask.

Asking about her grandmother was scary. She had not seen her grandmother. She knew that something bad, something serious, must be keeping Nancy away from seeing her granddaughter.

One day, Emily screwed up her courage. *Where's Grandma?*, she wanted to know. *What happened to Grandma?*

Mike and Amy told their little girl the truth. They said that the wreck had been a bad one, and that Emily's grandmother had died.

Once again, the tears streamed down Emily's face. Once again, she cried without making a sound.

When they were at the hospital together, Mike and Amy began each day the same way.

They visited the chapel at Riley, where they prayed, leaned on each other for strength and talked about what they had to do. They divided up the work confronting them, and struggled to meet the challenges before them.

As the weeks passed, it became more and more clear that Emily's spinal injury would not heal itself. She would not get out of her hospital bed and walk again without the help of a medical breakthrough. Things would never go back to the way they were for the Hunt family.

Amy knew their plan for her to return to teaching had dissolved. Almost all of her energy would have to be devoted to rebuilding her family and caring for her daughters.

Mike listened as the doctors told him what Emily's care would cost. They described the different kinds of wheelchairs, debated the merits of the various kinds of support stands to keep Emily upright and detailed the expenses of giving Emily the proper kind of nursing when she got home. They discussed the therapy the little girl would need during the coming years. They delineated the different educational aids she would require as she progressed through school.

When the doctors and the medical professionals got finished talking, the price tag was staggering—anywhere from 6 million dollars to 20 million dollars over the course of Emily's lifetime.

That was more, much more, than Mike's insurance would cover. It was more than Mike had saved or even could hope to earn. Emily's injury meant that the Hunt family was facing bankruptcy.

Mike and Amy talked for many hours about the disaster that was confronting them. Out of their discussions, a decision emerged and a plan of action took shape. They decided that they had to divide up the responsibilities before them.

Amy would tend more closely to the children. And Mike would try to find a way to keep his family from facing ruin.

Even little girls have a sense of dignity, a feeling that they are entitled to their own privacy.

Even when she was a baby, Emily had been reluctant to let anyone touch her. Often, she would let only three people hold her —her mother, her father and her grandmother. She was not a hugger or a kisser. She did not seek out and soak up attention the way Nikki, her more outgoing and aggressive twin, did. She did not want to be held by someone she did not know. Often, she did not even want to be held by those she did know. She liked—no, demanded—to have her own space.

That was one reason she took so much pride in being toilet-trained earlier than Nikki was. Some of her satisfaction stemmed from a sense of sibling rivalry, from achieving a milestone before her more boisterous twin did, but most of her sense of accomplishment came from something else.

Being toilet-trained meant that she had more control over her person. It meant that she no longer would have to wear diapers, that she would not be picked up, stripped and dabbed at. It meant that Emily would be allowed a little more of her own space.

The wreck and her battered spine tore away that hard-won personal space, tore away many of the steps Emily had taken toward becoming a big girl. That was hard for her to bear. Even harder for her to accept was the loss of the space she craved so much.

Because of the wreck, she had been put back in diapers. Nurses—strangers—came into her room, stripped her and changed her, just as if she were a baby again.

She reacted the only way a little girl with a strong sense of privacy could. When the nurses came in to change her, came in to dab at her as if she had never accomplished anything, Emily pretended to be asleep.

Asleep, she could deny that the violations of her much-cherished personal space were taking place. With eyes closed, she could pretend that this was all a game of scary make-believe. Asleep, she could keep the little girl's dignity she had worked so hard to acquire. Little girls cope the best way they can.

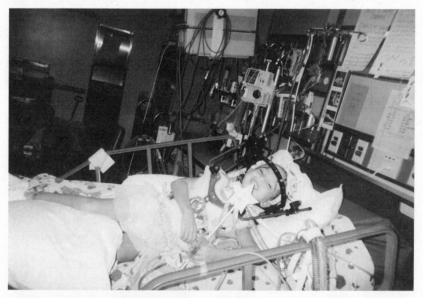

Emily smiles because she's wearing her first ballerina costume.

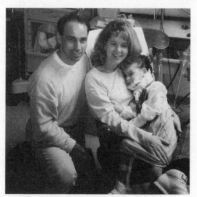

On the day Emily's head brace came off, Mike, Amy and Emily sit for a portrait. It was the first time Amy had been able to hold her daughter close since the wreck.

CHAPTER NINE

THE PLAN TO START BRINGING THE HUNT FAMILY BACK FROM ruin had its birth in a room at Methodist Hospital. Not long after the train wreck, Mike, Bud and Bud's son David Jones met in Bud's hospital room to plot how the family would respond to the tragedy that had gripped their family.

The initial planning, by necessity, was sketchy. None of them had ever expected to be in this position. They divided responsibilities. Bud would work to hold Old Indiana responsible for Nancy's death. Mike would labor to find a way to cover Emily's medical bills and keep his family from facing bankruptcy. David would help coordinate their efforts.

None of them realized how big the challenge was that they had set for themselves. But they all knew that they had no other choice. Nancy had died. Someone should pay for that. Emily might never walk again. At the very least, she deserved the best medical care available. Someone should be held responsible for that.

Quietly, somberly, the three men set about their work.

The job was bigger than they knew. The days and weeks following the wreck revealed that establishing responsibility—real responsibility—for Nancy's death and Emily's injuries would be no easy thing. The same quirk in Indiana law that made it impossible for Ern Hudson to make a criminal case against the owners of the Old Indiana amusement park also made it difficult for the family to pursue a civil suit.

The problem was the state's inspection history at the park. Because the state of Indiana said the train was safe to ride, the park's owners were free to shift the bulk of the responsibility onto the government and protect themselves from acknowledging liability for the damage they had done to everyone in Bud Jones' and Mike Hunt's families. The park carried insurance, of course, but only the rather paltry amount the state required, just 2 million dollars for all eight of the people who had been injured in the wreck.

Even if Emily had been able to collect all of the 2 million from the park's owners, her family still would have faced bankruptcy. Her care probably would require ten times that sum over the course of her life. In order to see that his daughter received the care that she needed, Mike would have had to thrust his family into poverty and keep it there.

So, Mike turned his attention to the state. Once again, he ran into a wall. Indiana law prevented him from launching a civil suit against the state for a private business's actions. That meant the state couldn't be held liable, either.

It was like macabre game of table tennis. When the Hunts tried to hold Old Indiana responsible for Emily's injuries, the amusement park swatted the ball over to the state. When the Hunts tried to hold the state responsible, state officials returned the serve back over to Old Indiana's side of the table. Even worse, if Mike started to complain about the state's negligence, Old Indiana's attorneys could use his words against him. They could argue that his complaint proved that the state was the party truly responsible for the accident, not them. That meant that anything Mike said about the state's responsibility made it more likely that Old Indiana would walk away from the wreck without being held accountable, and that his daughter would not get the help she needed. The game seemed to be rigged so the Hunts had to lose.

Mike consulted with his lawyers at the old, established Indianapolis firm of Bingham, Summers, Welsh and Spilman. They told him that his only hope lay with changing Indiana law. It wasn't a particularly shining hope. The change he would have to request would have to be retroactive; many legislators would oppose his proposal for just that reason. It would be a hard sell.

Mike called his father for advice. As always, Bob Hunt helped keep his son focused. The elder Hunt said that it sounded like Mike had a political problem and that he had better find a political solution.

Bob Hunt was right. It was a political problem, but that didn't make the challenge any less daunting. In order to get help for his family, Mike would have to shepherd a bill through the Indiana General Assembly. That was no small task.

The General Assembly was, in the words of one Indianapolis newspaper columnist, "the worst legislature in the country." The Indiana Legislature all too often was conservative in the worst sense of the word. The legislators generally resisted change regardless of whether the proposed change made sense or not. Often, they did so simply because they didn't like change.

There was a reason for that. Insiders acknowledged what was obvious to everyone, namely, that the General Assembly was driven by special interests. Indiana election laws were among the most lax in the United States. That meant that big corporations, insurance companies, utilities and other interest groups virtually could buy legislators.

Once they had made their purchases, the interests liked to keep an eye on the stock, so they sent lobbyists over to the Statehouse by the truckload. On any given day the legislature was in session, the halls outside the Indiana House of Representatives and the Indiana Senate would be clotted with lobbyists. The smoke from their cigarettes hovered like a small cloud around the rotunda, while the lobbyists buttonholed legislators and talked excitedly on their cellular phones.

It had always been that way. Years before, at the end of their sessions, the legislators had allowed the then dean of the Indiana political press corps, an *Indianapolis News* reporter named Ed Ziegner, to give a humorous address summarizing their accomplishments. One year, Ziegner told the lawmakers that they reminded him of a Little League baseball team, the kind of team that had its sponsor's names stitched onto the back of its uniforms. Unfortunately, Ziegner said, a baseball jersey wouldn't be big enough to list the names of all the sponsors for the average Indiana legislator. No, he said, the average Hoosier lawmaker would have to wear a cape to accommodate all the names of his or her sponsors—and even then there might not be enough room.

The Legislature was not a place where the little guy won. Money talked. Justice and fair play all too often took a walk.

At least two other factors complicated the job for Mike. The first was the nature of the argument he would have to make to the lawmakers; namely, that Emily had been injured through no fault of her own because the adults caring for her had placed their trust in the state's guarantee that the Old Indiana train was safe. In short, he was going to have to make a case that, as consumers, he and his family deserved some protection.

The problem was that Indiana had some of the weakest consumer protection laws in America. What few laws there were generally protected business owners from assuming any liability for their mistakes, regardless of how negligent those mistakes were.

Getting the Indiana Legislature to acknowledge that the state bore considerable responsibility for the damage done to Emily would test both the talent and the temperament of the most skilled politician.

Mike was no politician. That was the other factor that worked against him. Politics is a game of subtle codes, of feints and deliberate misdirection. For many politicians, particularly in the Indiana Legislature, the straightest distance between two lines is a zigzag. Most of the lawmakers ruling the House and the Senate in Indiana had the gift of implying one thing while truly meaning the exact opposite. They didn't lie, exactly, but they could be very skilled at getting a listener to leap to the wrong conclusion.

Misdirection was not Mike's style. He believed in a straight-ahead approach to solving most problems. He generally sat down and told the person across the table what he needed and what he could do. He took pride in being strikingly—even relentlessly—clear about his agenda.

Mike didn't figure that his approach would work well at the Statehouse. He figured that he had better get some help— that he had better find someone he could trust who understood how the political game was played and could help him map out a strategy. He needed someone to guide him through the dark corners of the political process. He needed to find an angel for his daughter.

He solved the problem the way he always had, by talking with people he knew he could trust. One Saturday afternoon, Mike called Tom Pence, an old friend from his graduate school days at Notre Dame. Mike asked Tom to put him in touch with Tom's older brother, Mike Pence. Tom said he would call his brother to see if he would be willing to help. Ten minutes later, Tom called back and said that his brother would be happy to help. He said his brother was at home and would be willing to talk at any time.

Mike Hunt didn't know it just then, but his daughter had found her angel.

At the time that Mike Hunt called him, Mike Pence had left the nitty-gritty of politics behind. He worked as a conservative radio talk show host and the moderator of a television political chat show.

In the late 1980s, though, Pence was one of the Republican Party's golden boys. Twice he ran for Congress against a well-entrenched incumbent, Democrat Phil Sharp. And twice Pence threw a scare into Sharp. The first time he came within a few percentage points of beating the incumbent. The second time he kept Sharp in a perpetual state of panic.

Pence's gift as a politician had been aggressiveness. He worried and harassed Sharp like a hunting dog that had treed its prey. His attacks could be cutting. In one of his television commercials, he accused Sharp of selling out America's interest to Middle Eastern oil barons. Sharp responded in kind, sending out his campaign staff members to argue that Pence was little more than a thug.

The two congressional campaigns created the impression that Pence was a right-wing attack dog. When Pence left the political world behind to become a TV and radio commentator, most observers expected him to be a bomb-thrower, a loud-mouth who specialized in invective.

Pence surprised them. He turned out to be a thoughtful analyst of public issues, a calm and even soft-spoken presence on the air waves. Other talk show hosts could specialize in bombast. Mike Pence carved out his niche by talking seriously about serious matters. His shows came to be seen as places where people could come to discuss solutions to pressing problems, not hurl insults.

That Saturday afternoon, Pence spent more than two hours on the phone with Mike Hunt. Mike explained to the one-time politician what he needed: a change in Indiana law that would allow the state to pay for his daughter's medical care. He said that he frankly didn't know anything about politics and didn't have a clue as to how to get started.

Pence had some concerns, he said. He wanted to know specifically what the Hunts wanted from the state, what they thought was right.

Mike told him the story. He explained that the state had inspected the ride and determined that it was safe, even though the investigation after the wreck showed that the park had been grossly negligent in maintaining the train. Worse, the fact that the state had certified the ride as safe made it all but impossible for the Hunts to sue the amusement park's owners. The state's role also protected the park's owners from criminal prosecution. Because the state was involved, Mike explained, Emily would endure a life of substandard medical care. Because the state was involved, Mike said, the Hunts were facing bankruptcy. Because the state was involved, the park's owners likely would walk away from a wreck they helped cause, a wreck that killed a wife, mother and grandmother and left a four-year-old girl paralyzed from the chest down.

Pence paused, and then said that this wasn't a question of money. It was a question of justice. Because the state hadn't done its job, Nancy Jones was dead and Emily likely would spend the rest of her life in a wheelchair. The very least the state owed Emily was good medical care. That meant the state had to acknowledge its responsibility for caring for her.

Getting that acknowledgment would involve a struggle. Pence took Mike through the process step-by-step. He told Mike that the greatest political asset the Hunts had was the affection and sympathy the public had for Emily. If Mike was going to be able to get Emily the help she needed, he would have to remind people of the wrong that had been done to her and show them that the state owed her something. To do that, Mike would have to use the media.

At the time of their conversation, Indiana was in the midst of a governor's race, one of the most hotly contested campaigns the state had ever seen. One candidate was Democrat Frank O'Bannon, an older, somewhat courtly man who was just finishing an eight-year-long tenure as lieutenant governor. The other was Indianapolis Mayor Stephen Goldsmith, one of the Republican Party's rising stars.

Most observers predicted that Goldsmith would win. During his five years as mayor of Indianapolis, he had become the darling of the conservative press. Goldsmith's major push was for privatization—the process of having private businesses perform public sector duties in the belief that business could do the work more efficiently and less expensively than government could. He pushed privatization constantly. *The Wall Street Journal* ran his op-ed pieces all the time. Right-wing think tanks like the Heritage Foundation and the Cato Institute touted him as a visionary. He appeared frequently on national news shows, where he came across as an energetic, almost hyperkinetic advocate for privatization.

O'Bannon, on the other hand, did not have a national reputation. Goldsmith seemed to be a young man in a hurry, an ambitious career politician on the verge of big things. Frank O'Bannon was more settled. A soft-spoken man in his middle sixties, O'Bannon talked slowly and avoided making grand pronouncements. Goldsmith cultivated the national media and won a big reputation as a political innovator. O'Bannon labored quietly in the Indiana Senate and then served in the thankless role of being the governor's second-in-command, but built along the way a network of enduring friendships with people who believed that Frank O'Bannon's word was one of the most secure bonds around. Goldsmith entered politics when he was in his twenties and never left. O'Bannon didn't run for public office until he had passed his fortieth birthday.

The truth was that O'Bannon did not have Goldsmith's vaulting ambition. O'Bannon wanted to be governor but not at the expense of everything else in his life. He believed in family. He told his confidantes that the governor's race was a win-win situation. Either he won the election and got to do a job he had always wanted, or he got to retire to his Southern Indiana hometown of Corydon where he could play with his grandchildren all the time. Neither option sounded all that bad to him.

During the summer, it had seemed likely that O'Bannon's grandchildren would have a lot of time to spend with their grandfather after election day. All polls gave Goldsmith a commanding lead of at least fifteen percentage points and sometimes even more.

As Labor Day passed, though, the race tightened up. Goldsmith made a series of mistakes, first by issuing a blatantly misleading campaign ad and then by dithering over his response as mayor to an incident in which a small mob of drunken Indianapolis police officers beat up several civilians.

Meanwhile, O'Bannon gained ground. His fundamental decency began to win people over. By late September the race was too close to call.

That left Mike Hunt with a dilemma. If he couldn't get the support of the incoming governor, any legislation he might suggest wouldn't stand a chance.

Mike's initial inclination was to place his bet with Goldsmith. After all, Nancy's death and Emily's injuries had taken place on the watch of O'Bannon's Democratic predecessor, Governor Evan Bayh. And Bayh had not overwhelmed the Hunt family with gestures of sympathy or support following the wreck.

Pence counseled Mike against placing all his chips with Goldsmith. If Mike bet on the wrong guy, any hope he had of getting a bill through the legislature would be gone. Even if he bet on the right guy, there was a good chance that the winner wouldn't remember or feel bound by any help the Hunts had given.

What Mike needed to do, Pence said, was try to get the two candidates on the record before the votes were counted. He recommended that Mike write letters to both candidates asking for their support for his bill. Then, to make sure that they responded to the letters, Mike should hold a press conference at which he announced that he had sent the letters and was awaiting the responses. That way, reporters from the newspapers and television stations would pressure Goldsmith and O'Bannon for their answers.

There was one other thing Mike needed to do, Pence said. The bill Mike wanted passed needed a name, something that reminded people of the wreck at the amusement park and the little girl who had been left seriously hurt by it. Mike should call his proposal "a Bill for Emily" or even "Emily's Bill," Pence said.

Mike liked the sound of "Emily's Bill." He thanked Pence for his help and hung up the phone, convinced that he had begun to see a way out of the disaster that had befallen his family.

He called Bingham Summers and told the attorneys that he had a plan. He said that he wanted to write letters to the gubernatorial candidates asking for help, hold a press conference to push them to respond and thus start a movement for something he planned to call "Emily's Bill."

The attorneys didn't quite know how to respond. They said that this was clearly something that needed to be planned out, so they set up a meeting right away.

When Mike got down to the law offices, he discovered that one of the attorneys already had begun working on implementing Mike's plan. If Mike was going to push for a bill in the Legislature, certain proprieties needed to be observed. That meant that Mike needed a sponsor for the legislation. The most likely candidate was Representative John Keeler, a doctrinaire conservative Republican who served Mike's district.

The attorney asked Keeler if he would be willing to carry the bill. Keeler turned the offer down flat. He was philosophically opposed to retroactive legislation, regardless of how serious the offense was that such a bill would attempt to correct.

Keeler's refusal only served to strengthen Mike's determination that Pence was right. The only way Emily was going to get the help she needed was if he pushed the process and made the politicians acknowledge the injury the state's negligence had inflicted on his daughter.

He wrote the letters, and sent them off by certified mail. Then he held his press conference, and announced that "Emily's Bill" was on its way.

Mike didn't have to wait long for the responses from the two candidates for governor. Pence had been right. The press conference had prodded them into responding.

Goldsmith's answer was almost dismissive, a polite expression of sympathy for the family's pain coupled with a rejec-

FRANK O'BANNON
LIEUTENANT GOVERNOR

STATE OF INDIANA
STATE CAPITOL
INDIANAPOLIS 46204

(317) 232-4545
FAX (317) 232-4788

October 24, 1996

Mr. Michael J. Hunt
8605 Allisonville Road, #121
Indianapolis, IN 46250

Dear Mr. Hunt,

Thank you for your letter. First, permit me to extend my sympathy to you and your family over the terrible tragedy you have suffered. Judy and I hope that your daughter, Emily, makes as much progress as is possible in recovering from her injuries.

I support the concept of the legislation you envision to provide relief to individuals who suffer catastrophic injuries. Obviously, the exact wording will have to be carefully drafted. However, I will try to be helpful to you as you seek to persuade the Indiana General Assembly of the need for this legislation. My suggestion would be for you to begin this process by contacting your legislators in the House and the Senate, if you have not already done this.

We will remember Emily in our thoughts and prayers.

Sincerely,

Frank O'Bannon

Frank O'Bannon
Lieutenant Governor

FOB:cc

This is the letter Frank O'Bannon sent Mike Hunt just before the 1996 election. Note the second paragraph's pledge of support.

tion of the plea for help.

O'Bannon's letter was something else entirely. It, too, began with an expression of sympathy, but then moved directly to a pledge to try to help the Hunt family in whatever way possible, including the passage of legislation.

O'Bannon's response gave Mike a lift. He began to believe that there was a chance he would be able to help his daughter.

He decided to repay the favor O'Bannon had done him. After the Old Indiana wreck, thousands of people had written, called or e-mailed the Hunt family, asking what they could do to help.

Mike began telling them that the answer was: Vote for Frank O'Bannon.

On Election Day, Frank O'Bannon beat Steve Goldsmith by a surprisingly comfortable margin.

Indiana had a new governor, and Mike Hunt began to feel that his family had a chance to crawl out of the pit the Old Indiana tragedy had pushed them into.

CHAPTER TEN

E VEN THOUGH HE HAD A PLEDGE OF SUPPORT FROM THE GOVER-nor-elect, Mike still needed help in the Legislature. Frank O'Bannon could say that he wanted to help the Hunts and that he was inclined to support Emily's Bill, but his support wouldn't mean much if no one introduced Emily's Bill in the Legislature.

O'Bannon couldn't introduce the bill. Only a member of the House or the Senate could, and the most likely candidate, John Keeler, the representative from Mike and Amy's district, already had said no. Mike had to find someone else to serve as his champion, and he had to find that person fast. Just two months separated Election Day and the opening of the General Assembly. If Mike couldn't find someone to carry the bill quickly, he would lose what little chance he had to help his daughter and save his family from bankruptcy.

Almost frantically, he started looking. Pretty soon, he found an unlikely champion.

Representative Candy Marendt, a Republican from the northwest side of Indianapolis, was not your typical politician. To be sure, she came to her office with a political pedigree. In the late 1960s, her father had served in the Indiana House of Representatives. At one time, he even chaired the House Judiciary Committee, on which Candy now served.

That bit of family history might have led some observers to believe that she was a standard-issue politician. She wasn't. Most members of the Indiana Legislature were lawyers. The relative few who weren't were insurance salesmen, small-town burghers or retired county sheriffs. Almost all of them belonged to a good-old-boy network.

When Candy was elected to the House in the 1994 Republican landslide, she was a divorced single mother who ran a day-care center out of her own home. She did not hide the fact that her life had had its ups and downs. When she was in college, she freely acknowledged, she had liked to party hard. She took a stab at law school, but dropped out. She took so much pride in her election she began wearing a pin that read "94," in honor of both the year she was elected and the House district she served, the 94th.

Most of her colleagues in the House calculated the political effect of their every utterance. They treated words as if they were land mines that could blow up on them at any time. Candy not only didn't speak that cautiously, she couldn't. Her emotions ran close to the surface of her being, and they often prodded her to push calculation aside. "I'll tell you exactly what I think," she said. "I don't know any other way."

Blonde, slender and, even though she was in her early forties, still as pretty as a high school cheerleader, she created a sharp contrast with the balding heads and pot bellies that marked most other members of the Legislature. She understood that her appearance could work against her, that her looks encouraged some people to treat her condescendingly.

"I know what a lot of people think about me," she told a reporter. "They look at me and think, Barbie's gone to the Statehouse."

The reporter asked her if it bothered her to know that some people dismissed her as a dumb blonde. She laughed. "No," she said, "because I know the truth. I know I'm not really a blonde and I know I'm not dumb."

During her first term in the House, she became a figure of some controversy. The Republican majority supported tort reform, a plan to put caps on the sums people could collect in civil law suits. Candy at first agreed with the idea of tort reform, but the more she heard from people who had been injured through negligence and incompetence, the more she reconsidered. Finally, she went to the speaker of the House, Paul Mannweiler, and asked to be released from her pledge to support her caucus's position.

It was a big step. Freshman members of the House rarely broke with their caucus's position on issues, and they never did so on issues as important to the caucus as tort reform was.

Opposing tort reform was something Candy felt she had to do, so she did it. She knew there would be consequences, and there were. Other members of her caucus began to whisper that she was a lightweight who couldn't be trusted.

Some of the whispering undoubtedly took hold. When Candy ran for re-election, she barely squeaked by, holding onto her seat by a mere eight-hundred votes in a race against an incredibly weak opponent.

Her narrow victory seemed to confirm the popular impression that she would not be a figure of much consequence in the House. Nevertheless, she was the representative Mike Hunt approached to carry the bill. He had tried with other people and been told no. Candy Marendt was his best hope.

Like everyone else in central Indiana, Candy knew about the amusement park tragedy. A mother of two children herself, she responded emotionally to Emily's plight.

That sense of connection to the tragedy grew stronger the more she learned about the wreck. She found out that one of the kids who came to her day-care business was one of Sarah Hunt's best friends. Somehow, knowing that just brought the tragedy of the wreck closer to home.

She met with Mike to discuss Emily's Bill. He talked with her earnestly, determinedly, about how much help Emily needed. How much help she deserved. He told Candy that he wanted the state to assume responsibility for its negligence, to retroactively remove its immunity from suit so he could get his little girl the medical care she needed.

As she listened to Mike talk, Candy arrived at two conclusions. The first was that she would help the Hunts in any way she could. They had done nothing to deserve the suffering that had been visited upon them. Decency demanded that she give them a hand.

She was under no illusions that agreeing to carry the bill would win her many friends at the Statehouse. Most members of the Legislature would react to the idea of retroactively changing the law the way John Keeler did. She would have to spend a lot of effort and energy just to get the bill heard in a committee meeting. If she managed to get the hearing, it was unlikely that the House would vote in favor of it. Nothing short of a miracle would push the bill through the more conservative Indiana Senate. Statehouse observers routinely referred to the Senate as the legislative killing field, the place bills went to die.

Candy's second conclusion was that Mike Hunt still didn't know just how big a task he had set for himself. Candy believed there was virtually no chance that Emily's Bill would ever become law. She could see, though, that Mike didn't realize that. She could see that he had no idea what he was up against.

In an odd way, the election had made Mike's job even bigger than it had been. The same voters who swept Frank O'Bannon into the governor's office also threw the House of Representatives into chaos. For the second time in the Legislature's history, the House was evenly divided: fifty Democrats and fifty Republicans. The split did two things. It gave each party enough votes to stop the other from passing a bill out of the chamber. And it created a huge incentive for both parties to posture and maneuver in the hopes of picking up in the next election that one extra seat that would create a clear majority.

That posturing and maneuvering generally meant that the Legislature only would be able to get around to passing the most important measures. At the top of the list was putting together a budget for the state. Just below the budget were education reform and tax reform. Emily's Bill was near the bottom. Still, Candy and Mike went through the steps. The bill they had begun to craft took its shape from Mike Pence's suggestion. Pence had argued that, at the very least, the state should never hurt an innocent party. This first version of Emily's Bill emphasized the Hunts' demand for justice. It called for the state to waive its immunity from suit, so that Mike would have a chance to prove that the state's negligence had contributed to his daughter's injuries. Even then, it emphasized that the Hunts wanted nothing more from the state than good medical care for their little girl.

Mike and Candy approached Representative Mark Kruzan, a Democrat from Bloomington, who agreed to co-sponsor the bill with Candy, provided he wasn't the lead author. He wasn't encouraging about the bill's chances. Then, Candy and Mike sought out a champion in the Senate.

They found one in Bob Hellmann, a Terre Haute Democrat who had just finished running a losing campaign for the U.S. Congress. Hellmann took a look at a synopsis of Emily's Bill and told Mike and Candy that one change would improve its chances from none to exceedingly slim. He proposed that it be altered to include toughening safety and insurance standards for amusement parks. That way, members of the Legislature might see it as a public safety measure rather than a special waiver for a single family.

Without that change, Hellmann said, Emily's Bill probably wouldn't even get a committee assignment, much less a hearing, in the Senate.

Before Emily's Bill went anywhere it had to get past one man, Representative Jesse Villalpando, the Democratic chair of the House Judiciary Committee. Villalpando was a machine politician, a product of the powerful Democratic Party organization in Lake County, the section of Indiana that was just south of Chicago.

Villalpando, thirty-seven, had been a member of the House for fourteen years. He was elected when he was twenty-three. Actually, "elected" wasn't exactly the way to describe the fashion in which he won his office.

He got tapped by the party while he was still a law student. He was just coming home from class one evening when he got a phone call from his mother. She asked how he was doing. He said, "Fine. Why are you asking?" She said, "Well, I just heard on the radio that you're running for the state Legislature."

Jesse paused for a second and then said that that was news to him. No one from the party had talked with him before pushing his name forward as a candidate.

Not that it mattered. Jesse always had been fascinated by politics and government. He wasn't going to say no to a chance to hold political office. Some of his interest he attributed to the fact that he had been born on the Fourth of July. And some of that fascination sprang from the knowledge that political maneuvering was as much a part of the atmosphere in Lake County as air and water. Almost everything was political in Lake County, and almost everything political flowed through the Democratic Party.

Certainly, politics came to define much of Jesse's life. He met his wife when she worked on one of his campaigns. They eventually had three children.

And Jesse's life settled into a comfortable routine. He had a solid law practice in Lake County and a strong career in the House of Representatives. Most elections he ran unopposed or virtually unopposed, which meant he didn't even have to campaign hard. Slowly, he became one of the more senior members of the Democratic caucus.

One of the rewards for seniority was a plum committee assignment. Jesse wanted to run the Judiciary Committee for two reasons. The first was that it was a prestige job, a chairmanship that attracted a lot of attention. That kind of attention couldn't hurt a politician who was still young enough to be considered a rising star. There were people at the Statehouse who touted Jesse as a possible candidate for attorney general at some point. Jesse didn't do much to encourage that sort of talk, but, then again, he didn't do much to discourage it, either.

The other reason Jesse wanted to be the Judiciary Committee chair was that the job would give him a prominent platform from which to push a cause dear to him, the reform of Indiana's wrongful death laws. The state's wrongful death statute was notorious. Tagged as "the worthless Hoosier law," it prevented the surviving relatives of any unmarried person over the age of eighteen who did not have children from suing if that person had been killed in an accident caused by negligence.

The insurance companies loved the wrongful death law. They argued that the issue was purely an economic one. Because no one depended on a single person for financial support, the loss caused by a wrongful death was solely an emotional one and no amount of money could eliminate a parent's or a sibling's grief.

The parents who had seen their adult children killed in senseless accidents hated the law. They contended that, in addition to preventing them from punishing the people who let their loved ones die, the law often frustrated their attempts to find out the circumstances of their children's deaths.

Jesse got involved in wrongful death when the father of a young man killed in a construction accident came to see him. The father's story moved Jesse, and he decided to try to reform the wrongful death law.

Thus began an annual ritual. Every year, Jesse introduced a bill to allow the surviving relatives of college-age and adult children who were victims of wrongful death to sue for damages. He produced the grieving parents, whose testimony often was delivered through tears.

Then, every year, the insurance industry lobbyists banded together to fight the bill. They showed up at committee hearings wearing expensive suits and carrying plushly crafted briefcases. While they testified, they glared at Jesse, a dark-haired, round-faced man who dressed in clothes that looked like they had been bought off the rack at Sears.

In the end, the outcome was always the same. The men in the expensive suits won.

At first, Jesse struggled to get his wrongful death bill out of the Judiciary Committee. Eventually, he did. Then, he struggled to get it out of the House. Eventually, he did. But there it always died. The Republicans in the Senate always refused to hear the bill. For ten years, Jesse pushed wrongful death reform. And for ten years he kept coming up a loser.

The long string of defeats left him frustrated. Few things in the Legislature mattered more to him than changing Indiana's wrongful death laws, but it didn't seem likely that he would ever get the job done.

Some observers thought that his long crusade to change the wrongful death laws made him a natural ally for Mike Hunt and Emily's Bill. Those observers were wrong.

Jesse was reluctant even to give Emily's Bill a hearing. Without a hearing, it would die.

Jesse's reluctance sprang from two sources.

The first was philosophical. He didn't believe that the state constitution allowed anything like Emily's Bill. He argued that the constitution prohibited state officials from passing a law that benefited only one person or family. The financial portions of Emily's Bill, Jesse argued, clearly were designed specifically to help the Hunt family.

Furthermore, Jesse didn't like the idea of retroactive changes in the law any more than John Keeler had. In Jesse's mind, going back in time to change the legal code was like altering the rules after the game was over. Doing so eroded the rule of law.

Those objections Mike might have been able to overcome in a discussion if he had had a chance to sit down with Jesse. But that sit-down wasn't likely to occur unless someone—the speaker of the House or the governor—put political pressure on Jesse to agree to the meeting.

But that was reason number two for Jesse's reluctance. As the legislative session was about to start, the political support Mike Hunt thought he had been promised by Governor O'Bannon suddenly seemed to have gone missing.

CHAPTER ELEVEN

I N THE WEEKS LEADING UP TO THE JANUARY OPENING OF THE legislative session, Mike started calling the governor-elect's office to find out what, if anything, was happening with Emily's Bill. Ever since he had received Frank O'Bannon's pledge of support just a few days before the election, Mike had tried to stay in touch.

The person he called most often was Bob Kovach, O'Bannon's top legislative aide. Kovach was an old-style political animal, a product of the St. Joseph County Democratic party machine who believed in old-fashioned meat-and-potatoes kind of legislation. He gloried in projecting a rough-and-tumble, man-of-the-earth kind of image. Every year, when winter began, he grew a bushy beard that came to look like an unmanicured shrub. When the first day of spring rolled around, he always shaved it off.

Kovach and O'Bannon were close. Once, when Kovach's life hit a rough patch, he even moved in with the O'Bannons.

Whenever Mike called Kovach to find out about Emily's Bill, the same exchange always took place.

"Is it on the radar screen, Bob?" Mike always asked.

"It's on the radar screen, Mike," Kovach always answered.

"Could you tell me where it is on the radar screen?"

"It's on the radar screen, Mike."

No matter how often Mike called to ask about the bill, he never got anything more than bland assurances that the governor-elect and his team still remembered him. Somehow, Mike didn't find that to be too reassuring.

There was a reason Mike couldn't pin down the O'Bannon team about the status of Emily's Bill. That reason? Emily's Bill was in trouble.

That trouble had several causes.

The first of them could be traced to the circumstances surrounding O'Bannon's pledge to help Emily. When Mike's letter arrived at O'Bannon headquarters, O'Bannon's team was in the full frenzy of trying to win a hotly contested statewide campaign. The decisions that get made in the last stages of a hard-fought political race generally get made one of three ways—on the fly, by the gut or in a hurry.

Because O'Bannon was exactly what his campaign presented him as being, a genuinely decent man, when Mike's letter came in, O'Bannon's natural inclinations encouraged him to help. Through no fault of her own a little girl had been left horribly injured. A family had been devastated. Who wouldn't want to lend a hand?

Once the passions of the campaign cooled, though, O'Bannon and his advisors took a closer look at both Emily's Bill and the promise the governor-elect had made. When the O'Bannon team took that look, they began to see some problems. They didn't know if the attempt to change the law retroactively was constitutional. They still wanted to do the decent thing, still wanted to help Emily, but they didn't quite know how. They quickly came to realize that helping her would be a much more complicated task than they had originally thought.

There were other complications, too. For much of that election year, no one gave Frank O'Bannon much chance of winning, so no one devoted much thought to what his legislative program might be. He might as well have been a cipher.

All that changed when he won.

After the votes were counted, expectations for O'Bannon's governorship began to climb dramatically. He went from being seen as a lovable loser to being touted as a legislative and political wizard.

There were two reasons for this transformation. The first was the improbable, come-from-behind nature of his victory. Anyone who could overcome that kind of lead while being outspent had to know he was doing. O'Bannon came to be perceived as a winner because he won when, by all rights, he shouldn't have.

The other reason for his image overhaul was even more complicated. O'Bannon's immediate predecessor as governor, Evan Bayh, had been just thirty-two years old when he took office. He had fair hair and finely sculpted features. He looked distressingly like a male model.

That was one strike against him. Another strike involved the circumstances of his election. Bayh's victory in 1988 ended twenty straight years of Republican sitting in the governor's chair. Many Republicans did not take kindly to seeing that streak end.

Nor did they have much respect for Bayh. One of their campaign slogans during the '88 gubernatorial race had been "don't send a Bayh to do a man's job," a thinly disguised jab at Bayh's youth.

The Republicans thought of Bayh as nothing more than a fair-haired boy who had climbed much too high much too fast. They were determined to send him tumbling.

The first two legislative sessions while Bayh was governor had been almost brutally contentious struggles for power. Neither side did much to seek compromise and, predictably, not much got done.

O'Bannon's election promised something different. Unlike Bayh, O'Bannon was a product of the legislative process. He had been a long-time member of the Indiana Senate before Bayh tapped him to serve as lieutenant governor. Then, as lieutenant governor, O'Bannon presided over the Senate, thus keeping his legislative contacts intact, even fresh.

When he became governor, many people began to predict that the legislative jams would disappear, that something resembling lawmaking miracles would take place. Even Republicans heaped praise on him. They said that Frank O'Bannon understood both the Legislature and the legislative process. He would be a governor who could get things done.

Lobbyists took such words to heart. Virtually every interest group in the Democratic Party lined up at O'Bannon's door to carol "Happy Days Are Here Again" and ask for the governor's blessings. Teachers wanted him to push for free school textbooks and more spending on schools. The union for the state's employees, whose wages hadn't kept pace with inflation during the Bayh years, wanted a pay raise. The mayors and other town leaders from the southern part of the state, where the residents tended to vote for Democrats, wanted a new interstate built to Evansville and more bridges across the Ohio River. Still other groups wanted tax cuts, more funding for police forces, greater spending on cities and better environmental controls.

Everyone, it seemed, wanted something. And everyone expected Frank O'Bannon to deliver because he was, in the words of one Republican senator, "a creature of the Legislature. He will get things done because he knows how the process works."

The crushing weight of these expectations almost overwhelmed O'Bannon's team. The governor-elect and all the people around him had just emerged from a bruising and exhausting campaign. Before they could catch their breath and regroup, they found that they were being asked to solve all the state's problems—and soon.

The big political problems—trotting out some budget priorities, keeping the teachers happy and reminding labor of the new governor's loyalty—the O'Bannon team took care of immediately.

Emily's Bill they didn't see as a big problem. There was time to deal with it. At the very least, the state could offer to offer a Medicaid waiver, which would lift some of the government caps on spending.

That ought to satisfy Mike Hunt, they figured.

They figured wrong. Mike knew about the Medicaid possibility, and he had discarded it. Accepting Medicaid would have made Emily in effect a ward of the state. That was bad enough from Mike's perspective, but two other considerations made the Medicaid option even worse.

The first was that he didn't think the waiver would provide Emily with the kind of care she needed. If Emily were to have a chance to have a satisfying life, she needed the best medical care available. Medicaid wouldn't provide that.

The second reason was that Mike thought the state owed Emily something more than perfunctory treatment. It was the state's involvement—its "inspection" of the train ride—that prevented him from being able to hold the owners of Old Indiana fully responsible for the damage they had done to his little girl. If the state prevented the Hunts from getting justice, the very least the state could do is make sure that Emily was able to see the best doctors. She deserved that much.

The first roadblock on the path to getting Emily's Bill passed was Jesse Villalpando. When the General Assembly opened for business in early January, Mike tried to get a meeting with Villalpando. He wanted an assurance that Villalpando, the chairman of the House Judiciary Committee, the committee to which Emily's Bill had been assigned, would hear the bill so the process could get started.

Villalpando couldn't give him that assurance. His reluctance to grant the bill a hearing stemmed from at least two sources.

He told reporters that he was troubled by the bill's retroactive nature. He said in interviews that, if the state went back in time to right this particular wrong, state officials would find it difficult not to do the same in other cases. Eventually, he said, the law itself would lose meaning.

Linked with that objection was the fact that he didn't think it was constitutional to pass a law that would specifically benefit one family. The Indiana Constitution banned such legislation. Villalpando could not see any other parties besides the Hunts who would be helped by Emily's Bill.

When he told reporters that he was reluctant to grant the bill a hearing, he cited his responsibility as chair of the Judiciary committee to protect the Indiana Constitution.

"I know there are people who say, 'Let the process work. Just give it a hearing and move it to the floor. Let the House kill it or the Senate kill it,' " Villalpando said. "But as chair of the Judiciary Committee I've got an obligation to make sure that the bills we hear meet a certain standard. And that standard is that they have to be constitutional."

That was the public reason for Villalpando's foot-dragging. The private reason was that Governor O'Bannon's staff needed time to figure out a way to fulfill his promise to help Emily. The new governor did not want to be in the position of seeming to turn a deaf ear to a young girl in a wheelchair. While O'Bannon's team searched for a way out of the predicament, Villalpando was supposed to hold the line for his governor and buy O'Bannon time.

Later, after much turmoil, Villalpando would insist that Emily's Bill always was going to be heard, that his reluctance to grant the bill a hearing had been part of a complicated dance of negotiations between the governor's office, the leadership in the House and the Hunt family.

That may have been true. If so, he was a good actor. At the time, it seemed as though his reluctance was genuine. When Candy Marendt tried to talk with him about Emily's Bill, Villalpando brushed her off. It was too early in the session, he said. There were too many other important matters to deal with first.

Then Mike began to call to see if he could get a meeting with Villalpando to discuss Emily's Bill. Mike approached the task of trying to win over Villalpando with the same sort of doggedness he had used as a rodeo rider. He grabbed hold and refused to let go.

His persistence annoyed Villalpando. After several phone

calls from Mike and more than a few attempts by Mike to talk with Villalpando in the hall outside the House chambers, the legislator finally talked with Candy Marendt about Emily's Bill.

"Get Michael Hunt to stop bugging me," Villalpando told Candy.

Thus began Michael Hunt's and Jesse Villalpando's duet of frustration. Before that duet ended, one man would have his career severely damaged and the other would know many sleepless nights.

They did not, could not, understand each other.

A casual observer who knew both men might have thought they would have much in common. They were about the same age—both in their mid-thirties. Both had been high school athletes, Mike as a football and baseball player and Villalpando as a swimmer. Both were married and devoted to their wives. Both were fathers who talked easily and lovingly about their children. Both were Catholics. And both had known early professional success, Villalpando in politics and Mike in business.

Powerful as these similarities were, their differences were even more pronounced. Some of the difference could even be seen in the way they moved. Mike always walked deliberately, as if he were giving great thought to every step. His head was almost always slightly lowered, and his often stern-looking dark brow would be ever so slightly furrowed. He paid attention to what was ahead of him.

Villalpando was a tall man with a round face and dark hair. When he walked, his arms almost flapped and his legs jutted out in a loose-jointed stride. No one could go through even a wide doorway at Jesse Villalpando's side. His stride took up too much room.

When he was in the midst of a serious conversation, Mike would become absolutely still. Not even his dark eyes would blink. Those eyes would look on to the person to whom he was speaking as if his attention had been machine-riveted into place. The effect could be almost disconcerting.

With Villalpando, the opposite was true. The more intense the conversation became, the more animated he got. Whether he talked or listened, his hands were in constant motion, pointing, gesturing, running over his face. His eyes rolled and his features shifted in a constant kaleidoscope of expressions. When he wanted to make point himself, he gently grabbed his listener by the shoulder, leaned close and started talking even faster.

That was the politician's way, of course. Most politicians see discussion as seduction, a chance to bring the listener over, an opportunity to win support, curry favor or pick up a vote.

The fact that Villalpando had been in politics for so long may have been one of the reasons he and Mike could not understand each other.

Because Villalpando was a product of one of America's last great old-fashioned political machines—the Lake County Democratic Party—he could not help but think about every piece of legislation the way a machine politician would. Politics was about deals. Everything was on the table and up for trading. No one got all or exactly what he or she wanted, but that was okay. Bartering was all part of the fun of politics.

With most issues, Villalpando's approach worked pretty well. Making laws generally is a matter of finding suitable compromises. The system rewards people who have the capacity to wheel and deal, who can juggle trade-offs.

Villalpando expected Mike to react the way professional lobbyists reacted to setbacks. Lobbyists generally came to the Statehouse with pie-in-the-sky proposals, bills they knew would be whittled away at in committee and on the floors of the House and Senate. The lobbyists came willing, even eager, to barter.

Mike couldn't, and didn't. Mike came to the Statehouse believing he was doing nothing less than fighting for his daughter's life and future. For that reason, he couldn't compromise.

To accept less than the best medical care available would be the same as saying that Emily didn't deserve to be healthy or happy. No father could say that about his child.

To let the political process water down the increased amusement park safety measures in Emily's Bill would be the same as saying that it was okay for Old Indiana to shatter his daughter's spine. No father could say that, either.

Mike thought that, at some point, Villalpando would understand that Mike couldn't treat his daughter's health as if it were a county building project. He couldn't make compromises where she was concerned. He couldn't ask for anything less than the best for her.

Not if he still wanted to call himself her father.

Mike thought that, because Villalpando was a father himself, he eventually would understand. Because Villalpando also had children, Mike thought he would come to realize that this wasn't a standard-issue political dust-up. It was a father's fight to protect his family.

But Villalpando couldn't understand that. The more frequently Mike called him or tried to talk with him in the hall outside the House chamber, the more angry and resentful Villalpando became. Other lobbyists could read signals and know when to come back with a lower offer. Why couldn't Mike Hunt?

Villalpando just didn't get it. His frustration came pouring out. One day, he was talking to a reporter about Emily's Bill. After the reporter finished inquiring about why Emily's Bill had yet to be heard, Villalpando turned the tables and began asking questions himself.

All of the questions were about Mike Hunt. What did Hunt want? Didn't he realize how the process was supposed to work?

The reporter, who had gotten to know Mike a little bit, tried to answer. Villalpando's mistake, the reporter argued, was in trying to see Mike as just another suit in the corridor outside the House. Mike wasn't a lobbyist—wasn't at the General Assembly to cut a deal for an interest group. He wasn't a political professional, and it would be impossible for Villalpando to understand him unless he accepted that.

Villalpando shook his head, vigorously. He started wagging his finger in the reporter's direction and said that the reporter had to be wrong. Mike Hunt was smart, Villalpando said. Hunt had gone to Notre Dame and gotten an MBA, Villalpando said. Hunt knew how to make deals. Hunt had to have an angle, Villalpando said. Now, what was it?

The reporter tried once again to explain. He said that Villalpando should try to imagine himself as Emily's father. He should try to picture one of his own children being hurt the way Emily had. He should try to imagine being helpless to stop his child from being hurt in that way: helpless to keep her from seeing her grandmother die and having her own spine broken. He should imagine a situation in which the only way he could really help his daughter was to see that she got the best medical care available and the satisfaction of knowing that some good had come of her tragedy—namely, that amusement parks would be safer.

That was how Villalpando could understand what Mike Hunt wanted, the reporter explained. Stop thinking of Mike as a lobbyist, the reporter said. Start thinking of him as a father.

As he listened, Villalpando compressed his lips and bobbed his head from side to side. Then he rolled his eyes and said, "That's too deep for me." And he walked away.

CHAPTER TWELVE

THE MONTH OF JANUARY, 1997, WAS ONE OF THE LONGEST AND most difficult of Mike Hunt's life. Every day, he drove down to the Statehouse and tried to find a way to get Emily's Bill heard. Almost everyone he talked to seemed polite and at least superficially sympathetic. But almost no one was willing to make a commitment to support Emily's Bill.

Every night he saw how much was riding on his efforts. Emily had come home from the hospital in late October. That was a good sign, but it didn't mean that her struggles or the Hunt family's troubles were over. Far from it. Emily required constant medical care. Every three hours, a nurse or a medical technician had to put a vacuum tube into Emily's tracheotomy that suctioned any obstructions out of her throat and lungs. Several times a day, the nurses pushed Emily through therapy sessions that a frightened little girl could not help but resent. At least three times a week, the nurses and one of Emily's parents took her to a nearby hospital for still more extensive therapy sessions.

Emily could not quite understand what had happened to her. She could not quite believe that her paralysis was anything other than temporary. When she spent too much time thinking about the accident or her grandmother or how much her life had changed, she grew sad.

Mike believed with a pilgrim's fervor that he could bring joy back to his daughter's life, provided he found the way to get her the right medical care. He came to see his struggle at the Statehouse as a kind of race. He knew how much care

Emily needed and how much that care cost. He also knew what the limits were on his insurance. By early January, Emily's care had consumed $600,000 of his one million-dollar policy. He looked at the numbers and knew that his family would not even make it through the year without help. If he could not find a way to make the state acknowledge its responsibility for his daughter's injuries, she would become little more than a ward of the state and the Hunts would be forced into a state of permanent bankruptcy. Generally, bankruptcy clears away one's debts and allows people to rebuild. In the Hunts' case, though, rebuilding their finances would have meant putting Emily's medical coverage in peril, a prospect Mike couldn't tolerate.

He faced a deadline. If he couldn't get a hearing for Emily's Bill in the House Judiciary Committee by February 27, the bill would die—and so would his family's chances of living a life marked by any kind of comfort. He had to find a way to make the state's officials see their duty by then, or he would lose the race.

It seemed as if he were trying to run in deep water, straining for all he was worth and only making the smallest bit of progress with each stride.

Day after day, he trudged around the Statehouse, talking, talking, talking, pushing, pushing, pushing. Each day, he thought he was making progress. He started out with a list. He knew his first goal was to get Emily's Bill out of the Judiciary Committee, so he began his quest by trying to talk to each of the fifteen committee members.

Every one of them said the same thing to him. "You've got my vote, Mike, when it gets heard," they would say.

Mike believed that that meant he was gaining ground. He did not know or understand the codes politicians use. The promises they were giving him were cheap ones, because none of the members of the Judiciary Committee believed that Emily's Bill ever would gain a hearing. After every conversation with a legislator, he walked away happy, not knowing that the pledge he had just collected was worthless.

Every night, he went home, spread his papers out on the kitchen table and tried to figure a way out of the impasse that confronted him. He told himself that there had to be a way to get the Judiciary Committee to hear Emily's Bill. He reassured himself that the governor would come through in the end. Sometimes, he even fell asleep at the table. Other times, he woke up in the middle of the night, consumed with a fear that he wouldn't be able to get Emily's Bill passed, and that he'd be able to take care of his daughter. That he would fail his family.

The worst part of it, the dread that never left him, was that he was overlooking something or forgetting something or neglecting to do something that might help his daughter. He knew that he could find a way to help his family survive this tragedy. But he also knew that he would have a hard time living with himself if his family suffered because of something he had failed to do or see.

Then, when morning came, he would go back to the Statehouse for another day of talking, another day of pushing.

Nothing seemed to come of it.

January drifted by without the slightest sign that Emily's Bill would be heard. Weeks passed without any indication that Jesse Villalpando would do anything about the bill. Governor O'Bannon refused to move. It seemed hopeless.

O'Bannon had other things to worry about besides Emily's Bill.

His administration did not exactly get off to a running start. He and his team seemed tentative, almost off-balance in their early days. Before his governorship was even a week old, there were whispers that all the stories about his legislative wizardry and political magic were nothing more than fairy tales.

Some of it wasn't his fault. From the first, O'Bannon dove head first into a strong current of bad luck.

His inauguration was an example. He and his handlers planned to make it one of the most memorable in Indiana history, a living history lesson. All Hoosier schoolchildren were required to study their state's history in the fourth grade. The inauguration of a governor, the O'Bannon team figured, would give those fourth-graders a chance to do more than study Indiana history. It would give them a chance to see Indiana history up close.

So, they issued a blanket invitation to attend the O'Bannon inaugural to the state's fourth-graders. They expected a few hundred, maybe a thousand to attend.

The fourth-graders surprised them. Hundreds of Indiana schools accepted the invitation. Thousands of fourth-graders planned to attend the inaugural.

The O'Bannon team reacted quickly. They began to see that, while having every nine or ten-year-old in Indiana descend on the Statehouse might present certain logistical problems, the public relations benefits could be immense. They closed off streets around the Statehouse so there would be space for the crowds and made arrangements for hundreds of school buses to find parking places. The O'Bannon administration began imagining that, following the swearing in, the state's TV stations and newspapers would be filled with accounts of Indiana's grandfatherly new governor playing host to thousands upon thousands of the state's children. It seemed too good to be true.

It was. As the inauguration drew near, the temperature started to drop. It kept on dropping. The weekend before the Monday swearing in, the mercury in the thermometer fell to below zero and stayed there. The governor's people prayed for a warming trend, but it didn't come.

When Monday morning rolled around, the temperature was three degrees below zero. The weather service predicted a high of nine degrees, but that would come late in the afternoon. Even then, the wind chill would be thirty degrees below zero.

School after school canceled. A few hundred fourth-graders showed up to listen to O'Bannon take the oath and make his speech, but the new governor's hopes of a media bonanza shattered in the cold. The stories in the newspaper and on television were about children getting frostbite.

It was an ill omen. Before the O'Bannon administration was even two weeks old, legislators in both parties and in both the House and Senate were muttering that the new governor wasn't giving clear directions and didn't seem to be up to the job.

The O'Bannon administration found itself struggling to stay alive politically. Too many people counted on them to help shape the budget and to make sure that the traditional Democratic Party interest groups got taken care of. Those were the priorities.

Emily's Bill wasn't.

Mike found himself feeling desperate as the deadline for hearing Emily's Bill drew near with no progress in sight. As January ended, he tried to start ratcheting up the pressure.

He started talking with greater vehemence to the media. He told reporters that he couldn't quite understand why the state didn't want to hear a bill that was designed to help a little girl and make amusement rides safer for children.

Some of the pressure seemed to pay off. Finally, after ducking him for weeks, Jesse Villalpando told a newspaper reporter that he planned to meet with Mike the following week.

After reading the story, Mike immediately sent Villalpando an e-mail message asking when the meeting could be arranged. Villalpando's office called Mike and said that Representative Villalpando would be willing to meet with Mike for fifteen minutes in the hallway outside the House chamber. Mike said that wouldn't work. He wanted to bring his lawyer along to answer any legal questions the Judiciary Committee chairman might have, and he wanted Villalpando to see all the documentation the Hunts had collected.

The dickering went on for a day or two. Finally, on February 5, a Wednesday, Mike went down to the Statehouse for a meeting with Jesse Villalpando. Villalpando kept Mike and his attorney waiting for much of the day, but finally came out to talk with them. The meeting lasted a half-hour.

Villalpando said that his primary objection to the bill was the way it changed the law retroactively. That wasn't constitutional, he argued. Mike's attorney answered that it was. The courts had allowed it. The Legislature once had raised its pay retroactively and the courts had upheld the Legislature for doing so.

Then they got to the heart of Mike's concern. He showed Villalpando pictures of Sarah and Emily taken right after the accident. Villalpando took long moments looking at the bruises on Sarah's face and the way that Emily seemed to be almost lashed into the head brace.

When Villalpando put the photos down, there were tears in his eyes.

Mike left the meeting thinking that his problems had been solved. The hearing would happen right away. But it didn't. Another week went by without a hearing. The bill seemed to be dead. Worse, the governor and his team appeared to be the ones trying to kill it.

Candy Marendt told him as much. Every session of the Legislature, bills were introduced in such a flood that almost no one could keep track of them until a few weeks into the session, when legislative services published a summary digest of all the bills before the House and Senate.

Emily's Bill—House Bill 1431, regarding amusement park safety—was one of the bills in the digest. But so was House Bill 1866, another bill on amusement park safety. It was an exact replica of Emily's Bill, minus the provisions to pay for Emily's medical care.

When Candy checked on House Bill 1866, she found that it had been introduced at the request of the O'Bannon administration as a way of getting around the governor's promise to support Emily's Bill. When Emily's Bill died without a hearing, the governor's team would be able to point to House Bill 1866 and say, "It's not our fault it didn't get heard. We tried, but we even had our bill that we couldn't get heard. That's just the way the process works."

Candy, as usual, had a blunter and more colorful way of describing the situation. "We've been screwed," she said when she called Mike to tell him about House Bill 1866.

The news left Mike in a quandary. He knew it was time to gamble, the moment to bet everything on one hand, but he really only had three cards to play.

When he first had conceived of Emily's Bill and talked with Mike Pence about it, Pence had told him that the media would drive the push for Emily's Bill. Everyone in Indiana was curious about Emily and would want to help her. When they found out about the governor's pledge to help Emily, they would wonder why the governor was taking so long to come to the rescue. Who deserved his help more—a hallway full of lobbyists or a four-year-old girl in a wheelchair who couldn't breathe on her own?

Mike had been trained as a businessman, and he thought the way a businessman does. In a business negotiation, a smart person warns his adversaries of the consequences of a particular course. *If you do this, I'll do this and it will blow the deal, so don't do it.*

Such warnings didn't work in politics. Politicians had to be shown the risk, had to actually feel some of the consequences, before they would move.

Mike felt that a crisis point had come. If he didn't do something quickly, Emily's Bill would die and his daughter would suffer. Mike couldn't bear the thought of that.

He called Mike Pence again and asked for advice. Pence told him that it was time to play two of his last three remaining cards. Those cards were the only way he could increase the pressure on the governor to act.

One card was Emily herself. He and Amy had prevented the media from getting too close to her. They had hoped to keep her privacy, which they knew she treasured, from being violated. Mike knew the newspapers and the TV stations wanted desperately to do stories on Emily. They wanted to get close to her, to see how she was bearing up. Mike had hoped to spare her those intrusions, but it didn't look as though he could. It was only by seeing Emily that people could see how desperately she needed help. It was only by seeing her that people could understand what the state had allowed the owners of the Old Indiana Family Fun-n-Water Park to do to a four-year-old child.

The other card was the letter from O'Bannon promising to help the Hunts. Mike hadn't released it to the media yet.

He had hoped he wouldn't have to allow reporters and cameras close to his naturally shy little girl. He also hoped that the governor would do the right thing without being pushed. But it hadn't happened. The governor wasn't moving. Pence told Mike to set up a chain of events.

The first was a story on Emily. Then Mike needed to have a meeting with Bob Kovach, the governor's top legislative aide. At that meeting, Mike had to tell Kovach that he was going to give the letter to the newspaper.

Then Mike had to give the letter to the newspaper.

That was the only way to make it seem as if Frank O'Bannon was ignoring a promise to a little girl in a wheelchair. If that didn't work, Mike's only remaining option would be to wheel Emily down to the Statehouse wearing a sign that read, "Why won't you hear my bill?" Mike didn't even want to think about that possibility, and how his very private daughter would react to crowds hovering over her while she sat in her wheelchair.

It might have to come to that. It seemed that Emily was the only one who could give Frank O'Bannon a shove.

The people in Central Indiana got their first glimpse of Emily on a TV newscast. One of the Indianapolis stations ran an ongoing feature called "Hope to Tell." The stories on "Hope to Tell" were supposed to be uplifting tales of courage and determination. The piece was touching and it provided people with the first real glimpse of what the wreck at Old Indiana had done to Emily, but it didn't do much—couldn't do much—to illustrate how desperate Mike's struggle was at the Statehouse.

To make that clear, the Hunts needed something more than a soft and fuzzy story on a TV station.

They needed a big story in a big newspaper. They got one.

Emily's story had been front-page news for *The Indianapolis Star* ever since the kiddie train jumped the tracks. *The Star* was the largest one in Indiana. Every day, roughly a quarter-million people bought the paper. Because most subscribers shared the paper with spouses, children and friends, the paper's actual reading circulation was more than a half-million. If Mike could make *The Star's* readers understand what had happened, he might be able to push Emily's Bill out of the committee.

The paper had done stories on Nancy's death, on how dangerously haphazard the state's maintenance of the ride had been, on the way that the criminal investigation had dead-ended and on how the Hunts hoped to pass Emily's Bill.

The paper also had done stories on Mike's struggle to get Emily's Bill heard, but without Emily those stories didn't seem to make an impact. Unless people could see her, it was hard for them to care about her.

Mike and Amy opened their home to a reporter and a photographer from *The Star*. The reporter spent several hours asking questions about the accident, about what their family was like and about Emily. The interview wasn't an easy thing for Mike and Amy to endure. The memories were still fresh. Recalling what it felt like to drive frantically from the mall to the hospital, recollecting the moment that Amy discovered her mother was dead and describing what Emily looked like when they first saw her after the wreck brought back a lot of hurt and fear.

Emily couldn't say much, of course, but she posed willingly, smilingly, for pictures.

The interview took place on a Wednesday. On Friday, Mike met with Kovach. He told Kovach that he was going to release the governor's letter to the newspaper. Kovach's face turned to stone.

Then Mike went and gave *The Star* reporter the governor's letter, almost as if he were dropping a bomb. The governor called him a few hours later.

O'Bannon said that the retroactive portion of the bill was the problem. If the state began trying to right one past wrong by changing the law retroactively, where it would stop? Other state inspections and institutions had been negligent. If the state allowed the Hunts an exception, state officials would be hard-pressed to deny other people the same option. The state would go broke.

The governor said that his administration would try to work out another solution. He asked Mike to remain patient. He told Mike that some offer would be forthcoming by Tuesday.

The governor's problem was no small one. As the whispers began to circulate around the Statehouse that he was trying to find a way to help the Hunts, legislators began to grumble.

If the governor caved on the retroactive portion of the bill, the floodgates would be opened, the lawmakers argued. Every citizen who had ever had any accident on a state-inspected site would come forward, and the state would have to play sugar daddy to them all. It would break the state budget and destroy the rule of law.

What this showed, the legislators contended, was that Frank O'Bannon—nice guy that he was—really wasn't up to being governor. Admittedly, it was tough to say no to a four-year-old girl in a wheelchair, but a governor's first duty was to protect the state's citizens and their resources. If O'Bannon wasn't up to holding that line, then he really didn't belong in the governor's office.

Whispers travel fast at the Indiana State Legislature. By that Friday night, the pressure on Frank O'Bannon had increased dramatically.

On Saturday, February 15, *The Star* published two stories about the Hunt family.

The main one ran on the front page, accompanied by a huge photo of a smiling Emily sitting in her wheelchair and playing dolls with her twin sister Nikki. The headline on the story was "Silent Cry Speaks Volumes," which was taken from its most affecting passage.

In that passage, Mike described what Emily and the family had endured in the hospital. He told the reporter how the tracheotomy prevented Emily from talking or indicating how much she hurt.

"The treatments were really painful, and the tears would just be streaming down her face, but we couldn't hear it. That was almost a blessing. It was hard enough watching her suffer like that, but hearing her cry would have been even more devastating. We were almost relieved that we couldn't. Now, of course, it's different. She has such a sweet voice and it really hurts not to hear it."

The story closed with a word picture describing how Emily wept without making a sound when she found out that her grandmother had died in the wreck.

The second story appeared on page two. It dealt with the specifics of Emily's Bill and the resistance the bill was meeting in the Legislature.

The story described, for the first time, how Mike had sought the help of both gubernatorial candidates. Mike had given *The Star* Frank O'Bannon's October 24 letter, and the paper printed the governor's promise. For the first time, people in Indiana read what the governor had said he would do:

> *I support the concept of the legislation you envision to provide relief to individuals who suffer catastrophic injuries. Obviously, the exact wording will have to be carefully drafted. However, I will try to be helpful to you as you seek to persuade the Indiana General Assembly of the need for this legislation.*

Later in the story, Jesse Villalpando explained that he had refused to grant a hearing to Emily's Bill because duty compelled him to hold the line.

"We have two concerns here," Villalpando said. "One is trying to take care of this little girl who has been horribly injured, and the other is making public policy for the whole state."

That was too much for Mike. To have the same politicians who were refusing to return his phone calls say they were trying to help his daughter struck him as hypocritical. In the story, he said as much. "These people don't say anything straight out and they don't listen," he told the paper.

He expressed his outrage over the governor's offer to grant Emily a medically fragile child's waiver of Medicaid requirements—an offer that he already had rejected.

"This does nothing for Emily. It provides, at most, $30,000 a year. Her medical bills are almost that each month. Why should she suffer for the state's negligence?"

The story concluded with Candy Marendt saying that Emily's Bill was dead, and that the O'Bannon administration had had a hand in killing it.

The two stories in *The Star* hit the Statehouse with almost explosive force.

As soon as the Saturday paper came out, the governor's office started getting calls. The number picked up on Sunday.

On Monday morning, the first real business day since the stories ran, the deluge accelerated. More calls. More letters. More demands for the governor to act.

The callers and letter writers all argued the same thing. A four-year-old girl shouldn't be made to suffer because the state failed to do its job. State officials shouldn't—couldn't—use legalistic arguments as an excuse to keep them from meeting the state's moral obligation to help Emily.

Justice demanded that they help her. Even more to the point, the callers—all voters—were demanding it, too.

As the calls and letters came in, the governor's people quickly realized that the Hunt family's problem suddenly had become an acute problem for them, too. Their wavering not only was causing whispering in the Legislature, it now was eroding public confidence in Frank O'Bannon's most potent political asset—the perception that he was a decent man.

The governor's staffers were both pragmatic and professional. They knew that they had to do something, somehow. They shifted Emily's Bill to one of the top spots on their priority list. And they went to work on finding a way to have the state help pay Emily's medical bills.

Governor O'Bannon wasn't the only politician who heard from people after the newspaper stories were published. Jesse Villalpando did, too.

The Monday after the stories appeared, he came back to the Statehouse to find his desk covered with phone messages and letters. He even began receiving e-mail communications. All the messages criticized him. One even called him "a moral amnesiac" for championing the cause of wrongful death reform while refusing to grant Emily's Bill a hearing.

The criticism battered Villalpando. He was not used to it. He had come to power from a district in which the Democratic Party was king. After the party first anointed him back in 1982, he never faced serious opposition. No one had ever attacked his record, questioned his reasoning or challenged his motives. He had never gotten bad press.

In fact, what press he had gotten had always been good. Because of wrongful death, he always had been depicted as a kind of white knight, a lonely warrior standing up to the big, all-powerful insurance companies.

Now, though, he found himself being portrayed as either a buffoon or a monster. The effect was disconcerting. He didn't want his family to see this. He didn't want his friends to see it.

But he knew the folks back home would know about it. The wires had picked up *The Star's* stories, and they were running all over the state.

Everyone back home in Lake County, Villalpando knew, would be hearing about the battle over Emily's Bill. Everyone would know what was being said about him.

The governor's phone call and the impact of the stories gave Mike hope. Maybe the fortress walls were beginning to crumble.

Mike felt some relief when he heard that the O'Bannon administration was at last trying to help his daughter. But the relief wasn't as profound as he had expected it would be.

He realized that, during the struggle to make the state honor its obligation to Emily, his thinking had begun to change. When he entered the fight for Emily's Bill, he had done so as a father trying to take care of his daughter and protect his family. His motivation—his obligation—had been to do what was best for his wife and his children.

The long hours he had spent down at the Statehouse, though, had made him aware of how hard it was for ordinary citizens to get their voices heard in the halls of power. He could recall every polite handshake and hurried dismissal from every legislator who treated him as if he were just another hustler on the make. He remembered every unreturned phone call, every brusque brush-off. He could call back every night he had spent at the kitchen table trying to figure out a way to get Emily the help she needed, all the while aware that his little girl, who once ran with the steps of a ballerina, was up in her room sleeping, unable to breathe on her own, her spine torn.

Mike knew that the politicians at the Statehouse hoped that a package of aid for Emily would be enough to make him pack up, go home and leave them alone. Part of him wanted to do just that. He did not like politics. He hated the insincerity and callousness of the political world. He loathed the way politicians said one thing when they really meant something else altogether. He wanted to be away from all of it. He wanted to be able to devote all his time and his energy to helping his family heal.

But he also knew that Emily's Bill was about something more than paying medical bills. He knew that if he didn't continue to push to make amusement parks safer, some other family would go through the same horror his had. Some other little girl would see her grandmother, her mother or her sister die. Some other parents would have to spend more than three months at a hospital, wondering, day after day, if their child would live. Some other father would have to wage the same desperate fight Mike had, just to care for his family.

Then there was Nancy. She had been killed because the state hadn't made sure that Old Indiana was safe. If Nancy's death was to have any meaning, that meaning had to come from her family's determination to make sure that no one else died the way she did. That no other family suffered as hers had.

Mike wanted to walk away, but he wasn't sure he could.

The governor had assured Mike that a solid offer of help would be coming no later than Tuesday afternoon. Tuesday came and went, though, with no word from O'Bannon.

On Wednesday, Mike decided another prompting was in order. He sent the governor an urgent message by courier. The message read:

"Per our telephone conversation on Friday, I expected to hear from you no later than yesterday regarding your decision to support Emily's Bill. As you know, time is running out.

"I am available all day today to discuss this issue….. After receiving your letter and listening to your inaugural address, I truly do not understand any hesitation to simply having a hearing and a vote on a bill that in essence:

1. *Makes amusement rides safer for children.*
2. *Increases insurance requirement in event of catastrophic events.*
3. *Provides for relief of medical costs to innocent victims who are injured as a result of willful and wanton misconduct by a state amusement ride inspector.*

"If I do not hear from you today, I can only assume that you do not intend to honor the commitment you made to my family in your letter dated October 24, 1996. Unfortunately I will be forced to seek an alternative method of securing a hearing for Emily's Bill."

The governor's answer came at 5:41 in the evening. It appeared in the form of a letter sent over a fax machine.

The governor's solution was little short of brilliant. In its most basic terms, the governor's proposal got around the retroactive portions of Emily's Bill by simply ignoring them. His plan called for the state just to assume that a trial had been held and the state had been found guilty. Once the question of responsibility had been determined, the challenge was no longer a constitutional one but a financial one. The state had to figure out how much care Emily would need.

The governor's people put it much more elegantly than that, of course. The O'Bannon letter began with an expression of sympathy for the Hunt family's suffering. Then there was a paragraph in which O'Bannon said that he agreed with the Hunts' push to make amusement rides safer.

The next two paragraphs argued that Emily's Bill was, in its original form, unconstitutional. The governor said he could not support changing Indiana law retroactively or creating a law designed to benefit only one family.

Then came the offer. The governor agreed to waive the state's immunity from claims of negligent inspection and award the Hunts $600,000 out of the state's tort claims fund. O'Bannon also said that he would allow Emily to claim the medically fragile child's waiver from Medicaid. The governor argued that the waiver would allow Emily to get the care she needed without forcing the Hunts to spend themselves into bankruptcy first.

And O'Bannon pledged to ask House Speaker John Gregg and Judiciary Committee Jesse Villalpando to hear the amusement park safety portions of Emily's Bill as soon as possible.

As soon as he had read and digested the governor's letter, Mike called the governor's office and asked for a meeting with the governor's people.

Over the next week, Mike dickered with the governor's staff. He asked how the administration arrived at the $600,000 figure.

The governor's people explained that there was a $300,000 cap on individual awards from the tort claims fund. The Hunts were being awarded the maximum for two people.

Mike countered by saying that there were five members of the Hunt family—and that no less than seven members of the Hunt-Jones family had been hurt in the Old Indiana wreck. Wouldn't $2.1 million or even $1.8 million be more appropriate?

The governor's team thought about it and came back with another offer: $1.5 million.

Then, in discussion with Mike, they put together a package of medical and educational aid programs for Emily. The package meant that she always would have the best care available.

The final agreement on the numbers took place on Wednesday, February 26, one day before the deadline for Emily's Bill to get a hearing. Mike had beat the deadline by a little more than twenty-four hours.

The moment the deal was struck, Mike sighed. His daughter would get the care she needed, the care she deserved. He had done his duty as a father. And everyone seemed to be happy.

Everyone was happy, except for Jesse Villalpando.

In the days after the newspaper stories appeared and the public pressure on him increased, he began telling people that he had delayed hearing Emily's Bill as part of a master strategy to force Governor O'Bannon and Mike Hunt to "negotiate."

He said that the people who criticized him didn't understand that he was really on the Hunts' side, that he wanted to get them the help they needed by pushing the governor to make an offer. People had to realize that he wasn't setting up a roadblock. "They didn't understand that all along this is what I wanted," Villalpando said when the deal was announced.

The governor denied that Villalpando had exerted any pressure on him. "I never felt any of that. I guess Jesse's been saying that because he's been vilified over the Internet," O'Bannon said at a press conference announcing the deal with the Hunts.

The complaints that Villalpando had been "vilified" over the Internet sprang from the e-mail messages he had received. He accused Mike Hunt of organizing a cyberspace smear campaign against him. Mike denied it. He hadn't told anyone to send e-mails to Villalpando, he said.

What he had done was appear on Mike Pence's radio

show and ask people to call the House Judiciary Committee Chairman and request that Emily's Bill be given a hearing.

Mike's denial didn't sway Villalpando. He was convinced that his reputation had been damaged by the Emily's Bill controversy, and he vowed to find a way to recover what he had lost. He asked Candy Marendt if she would surrender sponsorship of the bill to him.

She said she would. "I didn't care who got the credit for getting the bill passed, just so long as it got passed," she explained later.

Villalpando said he needed to be the author of the bill for a reason. "It's going to be my bill," he said. "I'm doing this because I was hurt politically by all of this back home, and they need to know what I did to help."

After the deal with the governor had been announced, Mike had a phone conversation with Mike Pence.

Pence congratulated Mike, and then suggested that Mike stay home with his family for the rest of the session. Emily had been taken care of, Pence said. That was the piece that most threatened the Hunt family. That was the part that Mike needed to take care of, and he had done so.

Pence said Mike should leave the other piece alone. Let the politicians battle about amusement park standards. That's what the politicians were there for—to wrangle back and forth in committee meetings and barter for votes.

As he listened, Mike thought of the other families who might have to go through what his had. He thought of how his daughter had looked in the hospital. He thought of how Amy still struggled to come to terms with her mother's death. He thought of how lonely Bud was. And he thought about Nancy.

"I can't do it," Mike said when Pence finished. "I have to see this thing through. I've got to make these rides safer." He owed that to Nancy and the rest of the family.

CHAPTER THIRTEEN

THE SOFT WARM GLOW OF GOOD FEELING GENERATED BY GOVERnor O'Bannon's settlement with the Hunt family lasted less than a day. Maybe it didn't even last that long.

Right after the governor announced the aid package for Emily, Jesse Villalpando publicly praised O'Bannon's act as "courageous." Privately, though, he told his colleagues and reporters that he wanted to find some means of turning the Emily's Bill controversy to his advantage. He wanted to discover a way to get a political benefit out of the publicity the bill had generated. He felt he deserved that, after having been "vilified over the Internet."

Villalpando thought he had figured out a way to make the attention work in his favor. He got the idea from House Speaker John Gregg, who suggested that Villalpando give Emily's Bill a hearing, but then amend the bill so it included all the wrongful death reforms he had wanted to pass for so long. That way, the Senate, which always had refused to grant wrongful death reform a hearing, would be standing in the path of the same juggernaut that hit Villalpando. The Republicans in the Senate would be the ones refusing to give a little girl in a wheelchair a hearing on her bill. They would be the ones getting the bad press, getting the calls and letters, getting all the criticism.

And, once again, Jesse Villalpando would be the good guy, a champion of wrongful death *and* the champion for little Emily Hunt, too. It was a beautiful dream.

All Villalpando needed to make it a reality was Mike Hunt's cooperation. Villalpando didn't mind exerting a little pressure to get that cooperation.

Mike got a phone call from Jesse Villalpando late on Wednesday, February 26. Villalpando told Mike that the Judiciary Committee would be holding a hearing the next morning at 9 AM. He wanted to meet with Mike beforehand to talk about Emily's Bill over breakfast.

The call boosted Mike's spirits. He thought that Villalpando finally had come around, that Villalpando finally had begun to see Emily's Bill with a father's eyes and understood that it was about making amusement parks safer for children and families. He looked forward to the breakfast.

When Mike got to the breakfast, though, the mood wasn't what he had expected. Villalpando had come accompanied by Tim Jeffers, one of Speaker Gregg's top aides. That was one troublesome sign.

The other was that Villalpando seemed to be nervous. He kept up a running stream of chatter, hands gesturing, face shifting from expression. None of Villalpando's conversation seemed to have anything to do with Emily's Bill.

Villalpando said he knew that Mike was a graduate of the Notre Dame business school. Notre Dame was a great school, Villalpando said. He always had been a fan of Notre Dame sports teams, he added. Then he recounted some of the great moments in Notre Dame sports history. This puzzled Mike for two reasons.

The first reason was that he didn't know how Villalpando had found out that he went to Notre Dame. That bit of personal information hadn't been in any of the stories about Emily, and Mike hadn't told anyone at the Statehouse where he went to school. The fact that Villalpando knew about Notre Dame indicated that someone had been checking up on Mike.

The second reason Mike found the Notre Dame sports history recital puzzling was that it was clear that Villalpando either was stalling or was working too hard to try to make a personal connection with Mike. People generally stalled or struggled to establish a rapport when they had bad news to deliver. Something clearly was up with Emily's Bill.

Finally, midway through yet another recounting of yet another great moment for the Fighting Irish, Mike decided to force the issue. He interrupted and said that he didn't think Villalpando had called this meeting just to talk about sports. Clearly, Villalpando had something he wanted to say about Emily's Bill. What was it? Villalpando stopped cold and looked at Jeffers.

Jeffers started talking. Then Villalpando joined in. They leaned in close to Mike, working him, trying to sell him. They said that there really wasn't any difference between HB 1431, Emily's Bill, and HB 1866, now that the governor had taken care of paying Emily's medical bills. Now that Mike's problem had been resolved, it was time for him to think about someone else. The system had done its part for the Hunts; now was the moment for the Hunts to give something back.

They talked about the way Nancy had died, about how it was a shame that Indiana didn't have tougher wrongful death laws. They wanted to change that, they said. They wanted to reform the wrongful death laws and they wanted Mike to help them. They needed his answer right away. If he wouldn't help them, they hinted, Villalpando wouldn't hear Emily's Bill that day. They would hear HB 1866, instead.

The pleas and the threats came all together in a jumble. The rush of words from Villalpando and Jeffers caught Mike off-guard. He didn't know quite what to make of what they were saying or exactly to respond.

He started by saying that he couldn't make the decision to support wrongful death reform at the table at that moment. The fight for Emily's Bill wasn't just his fight, he explained. It was a family fight. Before he could agree to make Emily's Bill a vehicle for anything more than amusement park safety, he would have to talk with Amy, with Bud, and with Amy's brother and sister. They all had suffered because of the Old Indiana tragedy and they all needed to sign off on any changes in Emily's Bill.

Villalpando and Jeffers made the push again. They told

him to think of how much Nancy's death had hurt his family. Then they asked him to think of all the other families who had lost loved ones, who had no way to hold someone accountable for the suffering they endured. Didn't Mike want to help those people? If he didn't want to help them, they said, they would just have to go ahead with HB 1866.

Mike started to say that he didn't know anything about wrongful death and that it would be irresponsible of him to promote something he didn't understand. Then it occurred to him that they needed him. Otherwise, they wouldn't have called the meeting in the first place. What they needed, he gathered, was his blessing.

He smiled and paused for a second, then said. "If you're asking me which bill I want heard, I'll make that really simple for you. I came here to support and testify in favor of Emily's Bill. If you give any other amusement park bill a hearing, I will oppose it. Is that clear enough?"

Villalpando and Jeffers took another run at Mike, working him, warning him, pleading with him. To no avail. The breakfast ended.

It was time to go to the Judiciary Committee meeting.

Most committee meetings in the Indiana Legislature take place in small rooms at the corners or in the basement of the Statehouse. The sites aren't supposed to be showplaces. They're supposed to be spots where a few people can sit and talk about bills that often are complicated.

For the Judiciary Committee meeting that morning, though, Villalpando had selected the chamber of the state's appellate court as the meeting site. It was a beautiful room with high ceilings and a wonderful old window that allowed plenty of natural light to shine into the room. The judge's bench was made from aged and polished wood.

The room was a perfect setting for television cameras. And the TV crews realized it. They had set up well before the meeting.

They needed to. The room was packed. Most Judiciary Committee meetings drew only a small handful of observers, most of them newspaper reporters or lobbyists directly concerned with a particular bill before the committee.

The interest in Emily's Bill had generated a crowd. Every chair was filled, and people stood along the walls. For a while, some tried to stand in the doorway. Then, Villalpando ordered that the door be closed. He didn't want any distractions, he said.

Mike was seated near the front of the gallery. Every few minutes before the committee meeting officially began, Villalpando came over to him to ask: *What's it going to be? Are you with us?*

Mike didn't answer. The more he thought about the way he had been treated at the breakfast meeting—the way he had been ambushed by Villalpando—the more angry he got. He struggled to keep his anger under control. This was not a time to blow up. Too much was riding on this hearing for him to allow Jesse Villalpando to goad him into doing something stupid.

The meeting started. Villalpando announced that the committee would be hearing HB 1431. Emily's Bill. He handed out the proposed amendments: the wrongful death reform amendments. There was a long silence while the Republicans on the committee read the amendments. When they looked up at Villalpando, their faces showed fury.

Candy Marendt came into the meeting a few minutes late. When she read the amendments, her heart dropped like a stone. She had surrendered sponsorship of Emily's Bill to Villalpando because she figured it was a small price to pay to get it passed. After Governor O'Bannon solved the bill's trickiest problem—the financial portion—she figured it would be easy to move the rest of Emily's Bill. Who wouldn't want to make amusement parks safer for children? If Jesse Villalpando wanted credit for making that happen, that was okay with her. She felt like she had done her duty.

When she had first entered the Legislature, her father, the old Judiciary Committee chairman, had warned never to give up sponsorship of a bill. Once a lawmaker took his or her name from a bill, he or she lost control of it. Anything could happen to it then. She realized she should have listened to her father.

When she finished reading the amendments, she looked up and caught the eye of John Keeler, the ranking Republican committee member. The look on Keeler's face said: *What the hell is going on here? What are you doing to us?*

By that time, Villalpando had started talking. As sponsor of the bill, he got to introduce it to the committee. Hearing him talk about Emily was more than Candy could take. She burst into tears, and ran out of the meeting.

Villalpando continued with his introduction. He said that the debate over Emily's Bill had focused a great deal of attention on the Legislature. Much of that attention had been negative. Much of it had been focused on him, he complained. "You might be forgiven for thinking that I had been wearing Bruno Magli shoes," Villalpando said, in a reference to the shoes O.J. Simpson supposedly had been wearing when he allegedly killed his ex-wife and another man.

That statement provoked another strong response. Representative Greg Porter, an African-American Democrat from Indianapolis, viewed Villalpando's comment as a racial insult, so he, too, backed away from the table. "These Bruno Maglis are out of here," he said, and left the room.

A minute later, Villalpando stopped talking for a moment. He wiped some tears away from his eyes. He apologized for the display of emotion. Later, he explained that he had begun to cry because he had found the criticism of his actions to be too painful.

When Villalpando finished with his opening remarks, he introduced Mike. Mike walked up to the lectern and microphone slowly. He stood there for a long moment while the TV cameras honed on him, then shook his head and frowned.

Finally, he said, "I guess I'm pretty confused about all of this."

He said that he had come to the Statehouse to help his daughter and to try to make amusement parks more safe for other families like his. Those parts of HB 1431 he could support without reservation, he said. He paused again. When he spoke, he said he didn't feel competent to talk about wrongful death. He had just learned about it this morning, and frankly didn't know what to say.

So, he said that he wanted to leave his endorsement of HB 1431 to the parts that focused on amusement park safety. With that, he walked away from the lectern and went back to his seat.

By the time Mike finished talking, the room had grown even more crowded. Somehow, the insurance industry lobbyists had learned that Villalpando had attached the wrongful death reforms onto Emily's Bill. They began pushing their way into the room to hear what was going on.

Mike was the only one to testify on Emily's Bill. The committee began to discuss the bill as soon as he finished. The Republicans, led by Keeler, began to question Villalpando sharply about adding the wrongful death amendments. Villalpando responded that he thought the amendments were a natural fit because "the grandmother, Nancy Jones, also died in the tragedy."

Keeler said that, because Nancy had been married, cases like hers wouldn't be affected by Villalpando's amendments. Villalpando said that was true, but he said that Nancy's death underlined a larger point. Her death showed how devastating such a loss could be to a family, particularly if it had been caused by negligence.

With that bit of skirmishing, the discussion came to a close. Democrats and Republicans glared at each other. From his seat in the gallery, Mike seethed. How could they take his daughter's bill and make it a political party favor?

The chair called for a vote on the amendments. The Republicans voted against all of the amendments. Every Democrat in attendance voted for the amendments. But, because of schedule conflicts, there weren't enough Democrats at the meeting to move the bill out of committee. Then Villalpando literally began to pull votes out of his pocket. He said that he had the proxy votes of all the Democrats who were not able to attend.

Keeler protested. He said that one time-honored tradition for the Judiciary Committee had been to allow members at least twenty-four hours to ponder amendments before they voted on them. Another tradition involved showing the amendments to all members at the same time.

Clearly, either some members had been shown these amendments earlier than others or some members of the committee would be voting in favor of amendments they hadn't even seen. Keeler said that either possibility violated the integrity of the committee and the process.

Villalpando waved his objections aside. The Republicans issued a formal protest to the vote. It was duly noted, but the amendments were adopted. Suddenly, Emily's Bill had been transformed into a wrongful death reform proposal.

That afternoon, the two sides of the Indiana House of Representatives wrestled furiously over Emily's Bill. The Republicans were furious. They were convinced that Jesse Villalpando had done something dishonorable. He had taken Candy Marendt's bill away from her without performing the basic courtesy of telling her what he intended to do with it. Several Republicans traditionally had voted to support Villalpando's wrongful death reforms. Now, though, they were determined to vote against his amended version of Emily's Bill when it reached the House floor that evening.

They even took the radical step of preparing their own minority committee report. The chances of the full House adopting a minority's version of the bill were slim at best. In the one-hundred seventy years of the Indiana Legislature's history, the House of Representatives had never adopted a minority committee report.

Preparing such a report, though, was the only way for them to register their outrage. They vowed, in the words of one Republican, "to fight this thing until the last dog dies."

Democrats also were angry, but their anger was less focused. On the one hand, they felt that Villalpando had been treated harshly during the process. They felt that Governor O'Bannon should have given him more credit for helping to make the financial settlement possible. And they felt that there was something spurious about the Republicans' cries of outrage. When the Republicans had run the House, high-handed power plays were the norm, not the exception, they argued.

Even so, they also were a little angry at Jesse Villalpando. They felt that Emily's Bill was the wrong issue for him to use as a political tool. They knew that most Hoosiers would be offended by an attempt to use a four-year-old quadriplegic as a political pawn. Villalpando had put them in an awkward, embarrassing position, right after the governor had rescued them from seeming to appear indifferent to Emily's suffering. They would defend Villalpando, but not without some muttering.

Without some sort of compromise, Emily's Bill would be in trouble all over again.

All afternoon, the leaders from both parties met, trying to hammer out a compromise, trying to find a way to make it seem as though the House wasn't playing games with children's safety. Every attempt failed. It looked as if Emily's Bill was in danger again.

To pass the Indiana House of Representatives, a bill has to be called for a reading three times. The first time it is read and then assigned to a committee. The committee works the bill over, makes whatever amendments it deems necessary and then returns the bill to the full House.

The second reading requires the full House to vote on all of the amendments the committee has adopted and whatever other amendments non-committee members may want to attach to the bills. Once the House has adopted or rejected all of the amendments, the bill moves on to third reading.

The third reading is the vote that ultimately decides whether a bill will be sent over to the Senate or not. It might seem as though the third reading were the most important part of the process because of that finality, but that isn't the reality. The second reading is where the bill gets shaped, and the third reading merely confirms whether or not the sculpting has been successful.

Around 8 PM, Villalpando asked for a second reading on HB 1431. The battle began anew, with the Republicans asking that the House consider their minority committee report.

Then Candy Marendt came to the front of the chamber. As she walked to the lectern in front of the Republican side, every eye in the chamber watched her. She moved slowly, as if she were trying to contain herself, keeping her own eyes down, as if lost in thought.

When she got before the mike, she took a moment to order her thoughts. Beginning to speak, she talked about how difficult it was sometimes to be in politics, how distasteful the process could be.

"Sometimes we all know down here that it isn't all that pretty," she said, holding back tears. "For Emily, let's leave this little four-year-old quadriplegic with a trach in who will probably be on a vent for the rest of her life—let's leave her out of this…. When a citizen comes and sees their government work like this, it's a disgrace to every single one of us."

Her frustration with the way Emily and her father had been treated came spilling out. She said that Villalpando had not been honest about the reason he wanted to sponsor Emily's Bill. She said that he hadn't even treated her with a minimal amount of courtesy.

Candy had not particularly wanted to carry Emily's Bill. The emotions surrounding tragedies involving children wore on her and left her feeling drained, but there had been no one else. She had took on Emily's Bill as a duty. She had told Mike at the beginning that he didn't have much chance at the Statehouse.

Somehow, though, Mike had managed to get the help Emily needed. He also appeared to have a chance to make amusement parks more safe for families. The thought that Jesse Villalpando might try to hijack Mike's gift to his daughter and the rest of the Hunt-Jones family infuriated her.

"The worst thing is that they tried to browbeat Emily's dad, poor Mike Hunt, into signing onto this wrongful death agenda," she said. When she returned to her seat, every Republican in the chamber leapt to give her a standing ovation. The Democrats sat and muttered.

The speeches went on. Accusations flew back and forth, while everyone waited for the other shot to be fired: Jesse Villalpando's response.

After almost an hour of debate, Villalpando was given the opportunity to close the discussion. He did not answer Candy's charges directly, other than to explain: "I didn't tell Representative Marendt about the wrongful death part because I felt I owed Mr. Hunt the courtesy of telling him first."

He argued that the wrongful death amendments worked well with the spirit of Emily's Bill. He asked the members to remember Nancy Jones. After Villalpando finished, Speaker Gregg opened the voting board. Quickly, the board began to light up. Every Republican voted for the minority committee report. Every Democrat voted against it.

One Democrat was missing. Representative Craig Fry had left the chamber, pleading a prior commitment. A House Democratic staff member was ordered to stand at Fry's desk to make sure that no one voted for him in his absence. Ironically, two months before, he had been the first member of the House Mike Hunt tried to lobby on behalf of his daughter.

The Republicans had won, 50-49. For the first time in the House's history, a minority committee report had been adopted.

The Democratic leadership had deliberately chosen a time when Fry would not be there to hold the vote. Democrats had decided to abandon Villalpando's wrongful death amendments. They had opted not to have a fight with a four-year-old girl in a wheelchair.

After the votes were counted, John Gregg talked to a group of reporters about the day's legislative battle. He told the journalists that Jesse Villalpando had been unfairly treated. "They're trying to say he was trying to do something political, but he wasn't," Gregg said.

Villalpando would have none of it. After the vote, he was angry—furious at the Republicans, at Marendt and at the Hunts. He accused them of being hypocrites. "The people who wanted Emily's Bill wanted the benefit of attacking me, but didn't want anything else. Now they've got a little bit coming back and they don't like it," he said.

He still had options, he muttered. If he didn't call the bill down for a third reading it would die. If the Republicans wanted to play rough, he could mix it up, too. Maybe he'd just kill Emily's Bill by refusing to call it for a third reading.

CHAPTER FOURTEEN

A LONG WEEKEND—FROM THURSDAY NIGHT TO TUESDAY— separated the second reading deadline from the last call for third readings. In politics, four days can be an eternity. Grudges can be forgotten. New alliances can be formed, old coalitions can fall apart.

In other circumstances, those four days might have been enough time for the tempers in the Indiana House of Representatives to cool, but they weren't.

Over that long weekend when February melted into March, both Democrats and Republicans seethed.

Republicans felt that the Democrats had taken advantage of the process by trying to link Emily's Bill with wrongful death reform. They felt that Jesse Villalpando had betrayed the House's code of honor by snatching Candy Marendt's bill away from her without telling her what he intended to do with it. And they felt that the Democrats had broken the rules of decency by trying to use the plight of a quadriplegic four-year-old as a lever to force the Senate to hear a bill it didn't want to hear.

They were not alone in their anger. The Democrats felt the unprecedented sting of having a majority committee report rejected and watching one of their own—Jesse Villalpando—have his reputation shredded before their eyes. They felt as though the Republicans had postured for partisan advantage, casting themselves as Emily Hunt's defenders when it had been Democrats, Frank O'Bannon and his staff, who had put together the financial package that made it possible for Emily's Bill even to be heard. They also could barely contain their fury toward Mike Hunt.

The Democrats in the House had come to see Mike Hunt as an operator, an evil agent determined to destroy them. Most of them had been locked inside in the Statehouse's stone walls for so long that they could not understand a way of life or a motivation that did not involve some measure of political ambition. The notion that a man's passion for change simply could be a desire to take care of his daughter and protect his family eluded them. They figured that Mike Hunt must have some angle, some hidden agenda.

So they muttered about the way he "manipulated the system" and about "how he was using his little girl." They complained about the way he kept pestering them, about the way he wouldn't read ordinary legislative signals and just go away. They whispered about the piles of money he was supposed to be making from his family's tragedy. They told anyone who would listen that Mike already had a TV movie deal locked up with Christopher Reeve, whom Mike had not yet even met. If it wasn't a movie deal, it was a book deal worth ten million, twenty million, thirty million … the figure grew with each new round of rumors.

Denials hit them and dissipated like a light rain. They would have none of it. Mike Hunt was the agent of their misfortune—one who was getting rich in the process of playing them for suckers—and they wouldn't have it. They just wouldn't have it. They'd show him.

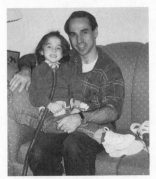

Emily sits on Mike's lap after coming home from the hospital. At that time, Emily needed a constant oxygen supply to stay alive.

The object of their fury knew he wasn't the most popular guy in Indiana state government, but he couldn't figure out exactly how things had turned so ugly.

What had started as something simple—a father's promise to his daughter—had turned into the biggest news story in the state of Indiana. When he first started going to the Statehouse, he figured that the financial piece of the Emily's Bill puzzle would be the most difficult to figure out. He expected a battle over that.

What he had not anticipated was a war over making amusement park rides safer for children. That, he figured, couldn't possibly be controversial. Who wouldn't want little kids to be safe? Weren't most of the legislators parents themselves? Didn't they want their own children to be safe?

Surely, Mike thought, the lawmakers eventually would realize that the governor had taken care of the hard part. They would stop squabbling and pass the rest of Emily's Bill, the easy part. The part everyone liked. Mike thought wrong.

When the House of Representatives opened on March 4, the Democratic leadership put out the word that Emily's Bill would be called some time after 11 pm, if it was going to be called at all. The wounds caused by the Thursday night bloodletting over the minority committee report and the wrongful death controversy still were raw.

Everyone in the House expected the third reading of the bill—if it even came—to generate even more fireworks.

The Thursday brouhaha had occurred early enough in the evening for the television stations to broadcast snippets of the squabbling on their 11 pm newscasts. The House leadership didn't want to have that happen again, so they planned a late-night vote.

That only piqued the media's curiosity. Reporters followed Jesse Villalpando around all day. They asked him, again and again, what he was going to do about Emily's Bill.

Every time, he told them the same thing. "Watch and see,"

he said.

Mike Hunt paced the hallway outside the House chamber. He had hoped that Emily's Bill would be called early. Then he heard that the bill wouldn't be called until late that night. He couldn't see any point in hanging around in the hall for another twelve hours. After all, he wasn't a lobbyist.

He decided to go to back to his office and do some work. Before he left, he gave Candy Marendt his cell phone number and asked her to call him if anything happened in regard to Emily's Bill. Then he left the Statehouse.

Early that morning, Mike and Amy had noticed that Emily was having trouble breathing. That wasn't all that unusual: she often struggled for breath. Her lungs, which had been damaged in the train wreck, never had really healed.

This was worse than normal, though. Even when Emily was fully awake, she labored to breathe. She took short, shallow rabbit breaths. She didn't seem to be able to get enough air.

They debated whether to take her to the hospital, but decided to wait. They had nurses in the house all day who could tell them if Emily's condition warranted hospitalization.

Amy watched Emily through the day. Emily's shortness of breath got more pronounced. Early in the afternoon, the nurse said that Emily needed to go to the hospital.

Amy tried to call Mike at the Statehouse, but couldn't reach him. Anxious to find him, she got a message to Candy Marendt. Candy called back.

Amy told her that Emily couldn't breathe and would be going to the hospital. She needed to know where Mike was. Did Candy have any idea? Candy said she thought Mike had gone back to his office. Mike got the call at the office, and rushed off to the hospital to meet his wife and daughter.

The doctors gave Mike and Amy some sobering news. Emily had a cold, a bacterial infection, the doctors explained. That wouldn't matter much to a healthy child, but Emily still was far from healthy. One of her lungs, the lung that had been injured in the train derailment, had never really healed. Now, under assault from the infection, that lung collapsed.

The doctors said Emily was in critical condition. They put her back on the ventilator, which represented a setback for her and her parents. Once Emily went on the ventilator, the process of weaning her off it would have to be started all over again, and that could take months.

Even more heartbreaking for Mike and Amy was some other news. The doctors said Emily was seriously dehydrated and needed more sustenance than she could take orally. They recommended a G-tube, a kind of feeding tube that pumped liquids directly into Emily's stomach. Inserting the G-tube required an incision.

The thought of their child having another hole cut in her gave Mike a chill and reduced Amy to tears.

At the Statehouse, the ill feeling over Emily's Bill festered. All afternoon and into the evening, the Democrats in the House tried to tell reporters about the big book or movie deal the Hunts had lined up. The whole thing was one giant hustle, they argued.

Such talk infuriated Candy Marendt. She often struggled to separate herself emotionally from the issues she championed, but at no time was that struggle more pronounced than when the issue involved children or children's care.

As the day drifted away and bill after bill got called, she grew more and more angry. To her way of thinking, the Democrats were posturing, playing political games to take care of one of their own, while a child fought to fill her lungs at a hospital and that little child's parents wondered and worried if their daughter would live or die.

She could hardly stand to look in the direction of Jesse Villalpando. Word drifted back to her about his threats not to call the bill for a third reading, and about his complaints that Mike Hunt had "victimized" him.

She couldn't stand it. The thought that, while Emily struggled to stay alive, the deadline for third readings might come and go without Villalpando calling Emily's Bill gnawed at her. She had to take action.

Candy told a reporter that Emily had been rushed to the hospital, and that the little girl was in critical condition. The news of Emily's condition raced through the House chamber like a grass fire. Tempers, which might have flickered out with more time, flared once again.

A little after 7 PM, Speaker Gregg recognized Jesse Villalpando. Villalpando called House Bill 1431 for a third reading.

When Villalpando sat down, Gregg opened the floor for discussion. In the back of the chamber, Candy Marendt raised her hand. Gregg recognized her.

Just as she had a few nights before, Candy started the long walk to the front of the chamber. Again, the chamber grew quiet.

Her speech on Thursday night had been one of the most dramatic moments the Indiana General Assembly had seen in years. Over the weekend, her political skills and stature had undergone a process of re-evaluation. Whereas she once had been considered a lightweight, even a ditz—"Barbie goes to the Statehouse," in her own estimation—that short speech had marked her as something else. A new spokeswoman for working mothers. A voice of conscience, of the outrage ordinary citizens felt when they saw folks like themselves chewed up by politics.

By speaking plainly and from the heart, she had created a new reputation for herself, and perhaps given herself a shot at a lasting political career.

On Thursday night, though, her outrage had been balanced by a sense of calculation. Honoring the House's traditions and rules, she had stopped short of attacking Jesse Villalpando personally or directly. She knew that maintaining an aura of affronted decency and dignity would make her point more effectively than any words could.

On this Tuesday night, however, that balance was gone. All she could think of was Emily in a hospital bed, struggling for breath, while Jesse Villalpando and his friends called Emily's parents little more than con artists.

When Candy reached the front of the chamber, she began her talk by saying what everyone in the House already knew—that Emily had been rushed to the hospital and was in critical condition.

Stillness settled over the chamber. The visitors' balcony was packed. Television cameras crowded the side balconies. No one moved. Everyone waited for Candy to continue.

She told the crowd that the Hunts had been unfairly maligned.

"There's no movie deal," she said, almost as if she were spitting. She tried to explain that Mike Hunt was just a father, just an ordinary man trying to take care of his family. The thought of Emily at the hospital overwhelmed her, and she paused.

The silence in the chamber grew heavier as Candy fought to control her emotions. Her voice breaking, she accused Jesse Villalpando of not telling the Hunts the truth and of treating them discourteously. She demanded that Villalpando sign a form she had prepared. The document called for Villalpando to surrender sponsorship of the bill so that she could reclaim it.

The howls of protests from the Democrats came immediately. Representative Michael Dvorak, a Northern Indiana Democrat, leapt to his feet, his face contorted with anger. A lawyer, he yelled, "Objection!" The speaker recognized him. "She is not speaking to the bill," Dvorak protested. "She is calling a member of the House indecent." Speaker Gregg told Candy that she had to confine her remarks to the merits of the bill.

Candy stood silent for a long moment. Somehow, she knew that she had overstepped, that she had lost control of the moment. Later, she would say that she had followed the best speech of her life, Thursday night's remarks, with the worst speech of her life. Worse, in doing so, she had surrendered the moral high ground.

She finished with a plea to Villalpando to give her back her bill. The Democrats protested again. Villalpando refused to look in her direction. He sat still and silent, his gaze focused resolutely on the front of the chamber.

Candy walked back from the front of the chamber to her seat in the back with tears in her eyes. She could not help but feel that she had failed Emily, and embarrassed herself in the process.

More speakers strode to the front of the chamber, none of them connected more than tangentially to Emily's Bill, but nothing they said registered with the crowd. Everyone waited for the other player, Jesse Villalpando, to speak.

Then John Gregg surprised the crowd. He surrendered the speaker's gavel so he could address the House. He wanted to explain something, he said.

It wasn't fair to blame Jesse Villalpando for linking wrongful death with Emily's Bill, Gregg said. The pairing had been his idea, Gregg said. He said it had seemed like a good idea, but it turned out that it wasn't.

Then it was time for Villalpando to speak. He said the controversy surrounding Emily's Bill had been difficult for him. He said that he had children the same age as Emily and that the thought of one of them being hurt the way she had was enough to devastate him.

He said that the battle over the pairing of Emily's Bill with wrongful death reform had obscured the most important fact—namely, that Emily's medical bills would be paid by the state and that a "constitutional bill" had emerged from the Judiciary Committee. He finished with a request that the House pass House Bill 1431, and sat down.

The speaker opened up the voting board. Within seconds, the green dots that symbolized a "yes" vote dominated the board. Emily's Bill had passed the House, 99-0.

Afterward, Jesse Villalpando sat at his seat and said to a colleague: "Can you imagine? What if I hadn't called the bill and the little girl had died?"

Reporters tracked Mike Hunt down at the hospital. He fielded their questions, calmly, patiently. Even though Emily still was listed in critical condition, now that she was being fully ventilated, the doctors had told him that she was out of serious danger. They had gotten to her in time.

The reporters wanted to know how Emily was. Mike told them that she was doing better, but that she probably would have to remain in the hospital for a while. Then the reporters peppered him with questions about the rumors that had circulated around the Statehouse all day. Had he signed a book deal? Was there going to be a movie?

As much out of relief as amusement, Mike laughed. "There is no book or movie deal," he said. "(The ABC-TV news show) *20/20* called the day before we made the agreement with the governor and said they were interested in doing a story on us, but they haven't gotten back to us. And we wouldn't get paid for it."

The reporters asked Mike how he felt now that Emily's Bill had passed the House of Representatives. Relieved, Mike said.

Later, after the interviews were finished, Mike shook his head. His little girl had almost died and had another hole cut into her flesh, and the reporters and politicians thought he was worried about a movie deal. What was with them? Didn't they have families?

Emily's Bill emerged from the House of Representative worse for the wear. In its original form, House Bill 1431 had been carefully crafted to meet the anticipated complaints that its demands for retroactive rewriting of the law were unconstitutional. The language was stiff, but precise.

After it passed through the Judiciary Committee and the adoption of the minority report, Emily's Bill became something else: a mess.

It had been rewritten hastily to accommodate the wrongful death reform language, and then just as hastily rewritten when that language was ripped out. There hadn't been time to tidy up or reconcile the changes. The House needed to vote in a hurry or the bill died.

The result was a bill that contained incomplete sentences and glaring grammatical errors. It made reference to sections that no longer were in the bill, and overlooked pieces that had been added. This new version of the bill made little sense and virtually guaranteed that the Indiana Senate also would have a battle over Emily's Bill.

There was one other change made to the bill. After the hub-bub had died down in the House, the Democratic and Republican leadership got together to try to resolve the dispute over the bill's sponsorship. Candy Marendt wanted sponsorship back and Jesse Villalpando did not want to give up control of the bill, particularly after he had been accused of virtually stealing it, so the leaders crafted a compromise.

Villalpando would retain sponsorship, but Candy's name would join his on the bill. And a third name would be added to it, that of Bloomington Democrat Mark Kruzan.

On the title page of the bill, Kruzan's name was inserted between Villalpando's and Candy's, almost as he had been placed there to keep the two of them from fighting.

CHAPTER FIFTEEN

THE HOUSE'S ADOPTION OF EMILY'S BILL MADE BIG NEWS IN Indiana. All across the state, newspapers and television newscasts did stories on the dramatic events in the House chamber.

The stories focused on the tensions within the House—the sparring between the Republicans and the Democrats, the dramatic speeches made by Candy Marendt and Jesse Villalpando, the sudden addition and equally sudden removal of the wrongful death reform language. The stories also honed in on the drama of Emily's rush to the hospital at the same moment that the House jousted over the bill bearing her name.

There was another theme, though, that began to emerge. Many of the stories began to focus on the improbable nature of the Emily's Bill triumph. The journalists described the Statehouse as a big, impersonal place, the fabled city hall that could not be beat. They wrote a story of a little guy who battled huge odds and won, overcoming much hardship and corruption in the process. They began to write their own Frank Capra-style political romance, with Mike Hunt as the Jimmy Stewart character. They saw the story as one with a happy ending. Justice had prevailed. Who could ask for more than that?

The supposed hero of these stories—Mike Hunt—couldn't see the House's adoption of Emily's Bill as a happy ending. It was a relief, another piece of the scrambled jigsaw puzzle he was trying to put back together. The puzzle was his family's life, the life they had had before the train derailed.

While everyone else in Indiana talked about the Hunt family's gains, the Hunts could only think about what they had lost.

Emily came home from the hospital after a stay of ten days, and the family's days settled into their strange, but increasingly familiar routine. Emily's therapy consumed the bulk of the day and much of her parents' attention.

The other girls for the most part had adjusted well to the damage the wreck at Old Indiana had done to their sister and their family. Sarah, in particular, showed an amazing sensitivity for a six-year-old. Whenever the girls played together, she took pains to make sure that Emily was involved. "Can you see, Emily?" she would ask. Or she would tell other children that Emily had to be included in whatever game they were playing. "Don't forget Emily," Sarah would say.

In other ways, though, the transition was a hard one. The girls had been caught up in something they had neither expected nor understood. Coping came hard.

Often, Sarah and Nicole would ask Mike or Amy when Emily was going to be able to get out of her wheelchair, as if their sister's paralysis was a game that should have ended by this time. They had difficulty accepting that anything bad could last for a long time.

They also resented the special attention Emily received. Their parents, their relatives, the nurses, friends and even strangers all focused on Emily. Reporters came to visit Emily, and Emily's picture appeared in the newspaper and on television. Everyone, it seemed, wanted to talk to Emily.

Nicole, in particular, had a hard time adjusting to Emily's celebrity. As Emily's twin, Nikki had been accustomed to being part of a matched set—and the more outgoing part of that set, at that. Nikki was more adventurous, less private and more extroverted than her twin. She smiled more easily and warmed to people more quickly than Emily did. Before the wreck, people generally noticed Nikki first. Now, they often didn't notice her at all. Getting used to being overlooked was not easy for her.

Difficult as the changes in the sisters' relationship were, the other change was even harder.

All three girls missed Nancy horribly. Their grandmother had been a constant presence in their lives, a warm and loving figure who took them out on special trips and never seemed to grow tired of talking with them or holding them. They could not understand how she could be gone.

Sarah understood death the best of the three. She was the oldest, and she had wept hard at Nancy's funeral because she understood that the wreck at Old Indiana meant her grandmother was gone for good.

Knowing something and accepting it, though, are two different things. There were times when Sarah would turn inward. Tears would come to her eyes, and her parents would know that she was thinking of her grandmother.

Nikki understood less about death than her older sister did. Sometimes, she grew confused and asked Mike or Amy when they were going to get to see Grandma again.

Her parents explained to her that her grandmother was in heaven, and that Nancy was with her all the time, but that was hard for a little girl to grasp. What a little girl like Nikki could grasp was that she missed her grandmother, and wanted to see her again.

Emily may have struggled with Nancy's death even more than her sisters. She and Nancy had enjoyed a special kind of closeness. Outside of Mike and Amy, Nancy had been the one person who could always reach Emily, always make her feel safe and comfortable. Nancy's death meant there was one less person to make Emily feel secure and one more reason to feel lonely, scared and vulnerable.

Nancy's death gave Amy reason to grieve, too. The grief came on at odd moments. Most of the time, her children kept Amy too busy to think about much more than the next task, the next responsibility she had to meet.

Emily, because of her injuries, required vast amounts of attention and energy. Amy also had to make sure that Sarah and Nikki felt loved and cared for. She also felt that she had to be a good daughter and help her father cope with his loss. And she had to be a wife to her husband.

Every moment of every day, it seemed, someone needed something from Amy. She wanted desperately to answer the call, to provide the strength and comfort her family needed so desperately. She wanted to be like her mother.

There were times, though, that the demands placed on her threatened to overwhelm Amy. At those times, the hunger to see her mother, to talk with Nancy once more, became something almost physical, like a gnawing at Amy's soul.

Amy always had felt close to her mother, but their relationship had deepened when Amy became a mother herself. Amy found it difficult to explain the change. They were still mother and daughter, but the fact that Amy had children of her own made them something else, too—friends, comrades, fellow travelers in a common cause.

Before the wreck, it had been a rare day when Amy did not talk to her mother at least twice. Outside of Mike, Nancy had been Amy's closest confidant and dearest adult companion. There was no question Amy could not ask Nancy. The knowledge that her mother was there, eager and available to pass on maternal wisdom and affection, made Amy feel safe, even blessed.

Now, though, Amy faced a challenge larger than she ever could have imagined. Every day asked more of her than she thought she could provide, but she didn't dare slip or stumble. Too many people depended on her. She had to stay strong for her children.

She needed Nancy more than ever, and longed to talk with her mother about how scared she was, about how worried she was about Emily, about how hard recovering from the wreck at Old Indiana was. She had a daughter's faith that a few words from her mother would make things better. But

Nancy was dead, and Amy felt her absence like an ache that never faded.

The months since the wreck had been hard ones for Bud. The holidays were the most difficult. Once upon a time, Thanksgiving and Christmas had been among Bud's favorite moments. Those holidays were a chance for him to gather his large and growing family close.

At such moments, he had believed that he was one of the most fortunate men on Earth. He had a bright, beautiful and loving wife, three children who made him proud to be a father, and a bevy of grandchildren whose presence made him feel born again. Because he loved his family, he loved his life.

But that was once upon a time. In some ways, time had frozen for him since August. He could not escape those moments at the park. Again and again, he saw his wife flying through the air and hitting the tree. Sometimes, he imagined that he heard the thump of her body against the wood.

Over and over, he relived the anxious effort of dragging himself toward Nancy's body. He could not forget placing his hand upon her leg, and thinking that he could feel the heat, the life, leaving her body.

And then there was Emily. Bud did not know how to act around Emily. Every time he saw her, the memories of that day, of those awful moments, gained new strength. He longed to reach out to her, to comfort her, to be her loving Grandpa, but something made that hard to do.

He could not help thinking that all this horror, all Emily's pain, could have been avoided if he had been a little bit smarter, if he had paid a little bit more attention to the vague warning signals he had felt at the park. Everyone else in the family told him that was ridiculous, that no one could have predicted the wreck, that he needed to give himself a break.

But he believed that a man's first duty was to protect. When the family got hurt, that meant the man had failed. That he, Bud, had failed.

For more than forty years, Nancy had been the person Bud turned to when he felt troubled, lonely or scared. Now he felt all three ways all the time, and she wasn't there to comfort him.

Mike Hunt read and watched the stories that cast him as a David who slew Goliath, as a little guy who won big, as a kind of romantic hero who had scored a great triumph.

Then he looked at his family. One daughter might never walk again. The other two probably never would feel completely safe again. His wife missed her mother the way a drowning person misses air. And his father-in-law reeled from the wreck like a man who had been hit so hard and so often that he could not remember where the blows came from or how hard they fell.

Some romance. Some triumph.

CHAPTER SIXTEEN

IT TAKES PERHAPS TWENTY SECONDS TO WALK FROM THE INDI-
ana House of Representatives to the Indiana Senate.
The two chambers sit just across the Rotunda from each other
on the third floor of the Statehouse, the House on the east
end and the Senate to the west. Most of the space between
the two chambers is open air, unconnected by a floor, to give
the Rotunda its majestic look and feel.

That open space might as well be a canyon separating two
tribes who sit on either side of the chasm. The Senate and the
House differ greatly in makeup, tempo and attitude. The pace
in the House is more sprightly and the attitude is more aggressive. The legislative dance in the House generally bounced
along to an up-tempo country-and-western beat, while the
action in the Senate moved in waltz time. The members of
the House loved to shout and carry on. The members of the
Senate saw a raised voice as a sign of weakness.

Since 1980 the Senate had been run by a team of four
men, now Republicans, all thirty-year veterans of the Legislature. They were President Pro Tempore Robert Garton, Majority Leader Joseph Harrison, Finance Committee Chairman
Lawrence Borst and Budget Subcommittee Chairman Morris
Mills. They called themselves "the ancient four."

By the time Emily's Bill moved over to the Senate, they
had been in power for seventeen years. In that time, the House
had seen no less than a half-dozen leadership changes. Four
different men had occupied the governor's chair. The ancient
four outlasted them all.

They were a formidable unit, in part because they saw
themselves as gatekeepers, the last defense against faddish

legislation and novel political enthusiasms. They were insulated from most traditional political pressures, because each man generally ran for re-election unopposed. Their power and clout gave them an immunity from public opinion that was remarkable. At the same time that both the national and state Republican parties fervently embraced the anti-abortion movement and made a politician's stand on abortion a litmus test for remaining in the party, all of the ancient four stubbornly remained pro-choice.

They thought of the Senate as a kind of legislative killing field, a place where bad or dangerous ideas came to die. They were old-line conservatives, the kind who believed in balanced budgets and no free hand-outs. They looked at society in almost Darwinian terms, and accepted that some pain and hardship had to be accepted as a cost for prosperity and progress. They saw themselves as tough-minded men, guardians of the public treasury, defenders who had to prevent more softhearted Hoosiers from spending themselves into bankruptcy.

They had the numbers to make their will known. The Republicans controlled the Senate with an overwhelming 31-19 majority. Whatever the ancient four didn't like generally didn't become law. In some ways, their power rivaled that of the governor. The Indiana Constitution gave the state's governor one of the weakest vetoes in the country. A simple majority in the Legislature could override the governor's objections. Nothing could override the ancient four's veto, once they had decided to oppose a measure.

If Emily's Bill were to have a chance of making it out of the Senate, Mike would have to find a way past the ancient four. The best place to start was with Garton. Mike called often, trying to get an appointment with the president pro tempore. Garton's schedule always seemed to be crowded. Finally, they talked by phone.

Once again, Mike told his family's story. He described his daughter's injuries, about the pain and suffering the wreck at Old Indiana had sent rippling through the family. Garton listened patiently.

When Mike finished talking, Garton said, in effect: *That's a moving story, but I'm not sure it justifies taking a nickel out of every Hoosier's pocket to pay for your troubles.*

Mike tried to tell Garton about the state's negligence in inspecting the ride and the responsibility the state bore for his family's tragedy. Again, Garton listened carefully, but refused to commit himself or the Senate to helping Emily's Bill. Mike could tell he would be difficult to persuade.

At the end of the conversation, Mike asked Garton how he should characterize this conversation when he talked with the media. Garton grew testy. He warned, in fact, he almost reprimanded, Mike about talking to reporters. He said they couldn't be trusted to get things right. Garton said that talking with the press wouldn't help Mike get Emily's Bill passed.

As he hung up the phone, Mike realized the Senate would be just as difficult a battlefield as the House had been.

When Emily's Bill passed out of the House of Representatives, it passed into the hands of two Senate co-sponsors, Democrat Bill Alexa and Republican Luke Kenley.

Of the two, Kenley was by far the most formidable. A balding, hulking man in his early fifties with a round face, an eighteen-inch neck and thick sloping shoulders, Kenley spoke in a drawl and liked to refer to himself as a small-town grocer.

He encouraged his Senate colleagues, particularly the women, whom he adopted in an almost brotherly fashion, to call him "no-neck" and make jokes about how ugly he was. He liked for people to think of him as slow-moving and slow-thinking.

They did so at their own peril. While Kenley did in fact run his family's grocery business in Noblesville, north and east of Indianapolis, he also had graduated near the top of his class at Harvard University Law School. Then, after he had joined the Army during the Vietnam War, he had finished at the very top of his class in officer candidate school.

Kenley didn't mention these things often, because he

liked for people, particularly opponents, to underestimate him. He enjoyed catching them off guard.

He had come to the Senate after a bruising campaign against a popular incumbent and had quickly established himself as a power in the Legislature. This was unusual. Normally, a new senator had to wait a term or two to get a plum committee assignment. Not Kenley. As soon as he was elected, he was named to the powerful Senate Finance Committee, and the word went out that Kenley was the heir to the throne.

If the ancient four were the old guard, Luke Kenley was the face of the future for the Indiana Senate.

Kenley got sponsorship of Emily's Bill for several reasons. Chief among them was his talent for defusing difficult political situations. Problems seemed to disappear when they landed on Luke Kenley's desk.

Behind his round, smiling face was a fearsome will to achieve and compete. He had a way of bringing people around without their even knowing it, because they thought that good old Luke was letting them have their way, when in fact he generally was letting them have his way.

Alexa was less daunting. The Senate Democrats in general were an ineffectual bunch, and Alexa was of the breed, taking direction from the caucus easily and not liking to take strong stands.

The Senate chieftains, the ancient four, did not like the kind of tumult that had surrounded the House's consideration and adoption of Emily's Bill. They put a premium on dignity. They did not want boisterous committee meetings with senators trading insults. They certainly did not want the Senate chamber to serve as a stage for the kind of melodrama that had marked the Emily's Bill battles on the House floor. Luke Kenley, they felt, could be trusted to preserve a certain decorum and keep things quiet.

Compared to the House's raucous Judiciary Committee hearing on Emily's Bill, the Senate Public Policy Committee meeting on Emily's Bill was a model of restraint.

The hearing took place in a regular and somewhat run-down meeting room, rather than the more TV-friendly state Supreme Court. There were no surprise announcements, no sudden and unexpected amendments, no hurried, tearful departures or resentful, muttered comments from committee members. Instead, there were only hushed voices as the senators talked about Emily's Bill.

That did not mean that Emily's Bill did not face serious opposition. That much became clear during the hearing. Mike showed up to testify, as did his brother-in-law David. Mike spoke briefly about the damage the wreck at Old Indiana had done to Emily and to the other members of his family. David told the committee that another Old Indiana patron had complained to the park's management. Bud testified, in his soft-spoken fashion, about how Old Indiana's negligence had cost him his life's partner, had deprived his children of their mother and had taken his grandchildren's grandmother away from them.

The committee listened respectfully, then voted, 10-0, to send Emily's Bill to the Senate floor. It seemed like a conclusive victory, but it wasn't. Even in the unanimous vote, there were signs of trouble for Emily's Bill.

The first inklings came from a pair of amendments the committee added to the bill. The first amendment called for amusement parks to keep their maintenance records at the park's main office, even if that office were far away from where the rides were and therefore well beyond the scrutiny of the park's patrons. The second amendment created a Regulated Amusement Device Safety Board that would include amusement park representatives. In effect, the amusement park owners would police themselves.

Bad as those two amendments were, it seemed likely that still worse ones would be coming when Emily's Bill reached the Senate floor for a second reading. The amusement park industry for the most part had stayed silent while Emily's Bill made its tumultuous journey through the House. The amusement park owners and operators reasoned that Emily's Bill was unlikely to make it through the lower chamber and they did not relish the prospect of a public fight with a child in a wheelchair, particularly if the fight was over a bill that wasn't going to become law, anyway.

Once Emily's Bill made it out of the House, though, the amusement park's reluctance to fight Emily's Bill faded away. The industry's lobbyists and strategists still did not want to have a public squabble with Emily, but they didn't need to. They started a quiet campaign of lobbying individual senators: calling the senators when they were back home in their districts, making quick visits to the office and huddling in the halls of the Statehouse for quick chats when the senators were on their way to lunch or dinner.

The quiet lobbying campaign quickly made an impact. During the committee meeting, several senators voiced concern that the increasing the amounts of insurance that amusement parks would have to carry would drive many small, Mom-and-Pop amusement companies out of business.

Those concerns gathered momentum when an insurance industry representative told the committee that no insurance company he knew of would write a policy without placing a limit on the size of the claim. The senators began to mutter that many small amusement operations would not be able to get insurance. Without insurance, they would be out of business.

Mike knew such talk signaled a serious threat for Emily's Bill. The Indiana Senate was first and foremost a pro-business chamber. It was largely because of the Senate that Indiana had some of the weakest worker's compensation laws in the country. Nothing could kill a bill's chances in the Senate faster than whispers that it would be bad for business.

The two changes to Emily's Bill the committee adopted,

allowing park owners to keep maintenance records away from the park and letting them police themselves, didn't please Mike, but he felt that he could live with those alterations.

Lowering the insurance requirements was something else all together. Mike couldn't accept that, because accepting it would mean that somewhere, some time, another family would be left in his family's situation. Another father would have to choose between bankruptcy and paying his child's medical bills. Another little boy or girl would face a life diminished because his or her family couldn't afford good medical care.

Mike heard the whispers about the insurance requirements being bad for business, and feared that Emily's Bill was in trouble once again.

Those fears became reality when Emily's Bill reached the Senate floor on second reading. Senator Alexa offered three amendments. The first two weren't controversial. They called for amusement parks to carry at least one million of insurance for each individual accident and five million for a large, multiple-person accident or repeated accidents during the course of a year.

The third amendment, though, hit Mike with the force of a slap in the face. It called for amusement companies that deal primarily with kiddie rides to only have to carry $500,000 of insurance per occurrence and two million for a multiple-person accident or repeated accidents. Alexa said he offered the amendment because several amusement companies that provided rides for county fairs had told him that higher insurance requirements would force them to go out of business.

He hadn't bothered to ask if they should even be in business if they couldn't guarantee that people would not be killed or maimed on their rides, or at least that an injured person's medical bills would be paid if one of their rides malfunctioned.

Not many other senators asked that question, either. The amendment passed, 38-10.

Mike wasted no time in blasting it to the press. He said that lowering the insurance requirements on kiddie rides made no sense. "That's too low," he told a reporter. "My family is living proof of that. Emily is living proof that two million is not enough."

He couldn't believe that the Senate was about to make the same mistake as the House. "You would think that they'd learn that everyone who fools around with this ends up looking foolish," he fumed.

The amendments to Emily's Bill left Mike with an awkward choice. If he made too much noise about his displeasure, the bill might not get a third reading in the Senate. That would effectively kill it, which meant that amusement park rides in the state wouldn't be any safer than they were when he started.

He couldn't have that. So, he swallowed his anger, and told everyone in sight that, while he didn't like the amendments, he still supported the bill.

Then he began planning to go to war for Emily's Bill one more time. As he prepared for the fight, Mike discovered that he had a surprising new ally: Jesse Villalpando.

CHAPTER SEVENTEEN

IN THEORY, A BILL BECOMES LAW IN INDIANA BECAUSE THE TWO houses of the Legislature agree that it is a good idea and adopt exactly the same bill with exactly the same language.

Often, that is the way the legislative process works. Generally, though, the bills that move that smoothly through the system are not bills about which people care a great deal. The bills that make it through the committee process in both the House and the Senate and then emerge from the floors of both chambers without alteration most often do not generate much controversy.

Emily's Bill had generated a lot of controversy. The struggle to get the bill passed, the conflict between Jesse Villalpando and Candy Marendt, the two televised showdowns on the House floor and the emergence of Mike Hunt as a Frank-Capra-like hero had made Emily's Bill a big story. A lot of people had an interest in either helping Emily's Bill to become law or preventing it from becoming an effective law.

In the nearly four months that the Legislature had been in session, Emily's Bill had been twisted and transformed again and again. The bill that emerged from the Senate little resembled the one the House had passed. That meant that Emily's Bill faced yet another step in the legislative process: a conference committee.

The conference committee process seems simple. A Republican and a Democrat from the House of Representatives and a Republican and a Democrat from the Senate sit down to work out their differences. Once they reach an agreement and hammer out new language that is acceptable to everyone, the representatives and senators take the new version back to their respective chambers for a new vote. If the Senate and the House vote in favor of the new language, the amended bill moves onto the governor, who signs it into law.

If, however, the conference committee can't agree on new language or either chamber the Legislature rejects the amended bill, it dies. Because conference committees meet at the very end of the legislative session, that generally means that the bill's sponsors will have to wait at least another year to try again.

There were people who did that—who brought good causes back to the Statehouse year after year after year without ever seeing their bills become law. Mike Hunt did not want to be one of those people.

In the case of Emily's Bill, Mike knew that there probably wouldn't be a next year. He had learned enough about the political process to understand that the longer he waited to pass Emily's Bill the less chance he would have to see it become law. People cared about amusement park safety at the moment because the wreck at Old Indiana and the pictures of Emily in her wheelchair were still fresh in their minds. In a year's time, some new tragedy and some new cause would occupy the public's attention.

The politicians would stop caring just as soon as the public did. They had not been eager to deal with Emily's Bill from the beginning. Now that the amusement park industry had roused itself to oppose the bill, the senators and representatives were even less enthusiastic. If Emily's Bill failed and Mike tried to come back a year later, he could look forward to an even more difficult challenge he had faced in getting the bill heard this time around: more unreturned phone calls, less courtesy and communication.

That was the danger for Mike and Emily's Bill. It had to be this year or no year. If he failed, he failed for good. That also was his strength.

Because the public still remembered the wreck and still could see the images of Emily in her wheelchair, Mike still could exert a great deal of political pressure on the members. That is why he decided to go for broke, to demand that the Legislature adopt a bill that met his standards or face the consequences of having him, Emily Hunt's father, refuse to endorse Emily's Bill.

To make his threat credible, Mike needed an ally. And he found an unlikely one.

The controversy over Emily's Bill in the House had left Jesse Villalpando shaken. For years, he had seen himself as a gallant warrior fighting the good fight, carrying the standard for families who had lost children in horrible accidents and had nowhere to run for help. He believed that the public always had seen him that way, too. Emily's Bill had changed that.

Suddenly, he found himself depicted as a man who was denying aid to a little girl who likely would never walk again. He found himself accused of denying her father a chance at a fair hearing, and he read stories in the newspaper that criticized him for manipulating the political process for his own ends.

Villalpando felt pounded by the criticism, the accusations and the portraits of him as a cruel man. "Most legislative battles I shrug off," he told a reporter. "But not this one. This one got to me. It hurt."

When Emily's Bill made it out of the Senate in its altered form and got sent to a conference committee, Villalpando knew that he would have another chance to make things right. He wanted to remind people that he was not a heartless man, that he had worked for many victims of accidents as horrible as Emily's for many years, to be Emily's champion.

Four people sat on the Emily's Bill conference committee: Luke Kenley and William Alexa from the Senate and Jesse Villalpando and Brent Steele from the House. Steele, a thoughtful, bearded Republican with impeccable conservative credentials, sat in the place of Candy Marendt, who did not want to work on Emily's Bill with Jesse Villalpando again.

The members of the conference committee met at a folding table in a ramshackle room in the basement of the Statehouse hearing testimony. Mike spoke briefly in favor of the bill and asked that the committee consider reinstating the higher insurance requirements for kiddie rides. Then several people from the amusement park and insurance industries testified that Emily's Bill would do damage to business.

The members of the conference committee sat in silence for a moment, then they began to speak. Luke Kenley said that the insurance requirements had been an obstacle to getting the bill passed in the Senate in the first place and that increasing them would probably doom the bill's chances.

Jesse Villalpando immediately chimed in that he really wanted to get a bill passed. After all the work the House and Senate had done and all the controversy, it was really important for the public to see that something had been done, he said.

Kenley rolled his eyes. In a few short sentences, Villalpando had just traded away his negotiating position. He had said that he would accept just about any bill to get one passed.

For a moment, Mike shared Kenley's disbelief. But he quickly came to realize that Villalpando's determination not to get on the wrong side of Emily Hunt again gave Mike some leverage. Because Villalpando was the sponsor of Emily's Bill, he could withdraw it from consideration at any time.

If Mike could persuade Villalpando to threaten to withdraw the bill because the Senate was being obstinate, he'd be in a high stakes game of chicken with the amusement park industry. He was willing to bet that he would win.

Villalpando asked the conference committee to accept higher insurance requirements on kiddie rides. He said they were necessary. Kenley didn't sound encouraging. "I might have a problem with my caucus," he said.

The four members of the conference committee agreed to the higher insurance requirements for kiddie rides, but both Kenley and Alexa said they weren't optimistic that their caucuses would agree to the increases. The meeting broke up with a feeling that not much had been resolved.

The tentative agreement broke down almost as soon as the meeting ended.

Kenley and Alexa emerged from meetings with their caucuses saying that they could not sign the conference committee report as long as the higher insurance requirements were in place.

"My caucus decided they'd prefer to go with the lower number. The feeling was that it's easier to go up later than to come down," Kenley told a reporter.

Alexa put it even more bluntly. "The caucus wasn't comfortable with the one million figure and didn't want me to sign," he said. That left Mike just where he had feared he would be, in the middle of a showdown with the Senate and the amusement park industry. He felt that it was time to use all the weapons at his disposal.

First, he talked with Jesse Villalpando. He told him that he could not endorse Emily's Bill if the lower insurance requirements were in place. He said he would support him if he withdrew the bill from consideration and put the blame for the withdrawal on the Senate.

Villalpando seemed stunned by the turn of events. He kept asking Mike if that was what he really wanted to do. Almost hesitantly, he voiced some concerns about throwing away months of hard work and, indirectly, he said he was worried about seeming to be the guy who killed Emily's Bill.

Mike assured him that this was what the Hunt family wanted. He told Villalpando that his daughter's predicament demonstrated that $500,000 per accident wasn't enough to insure that children would be safe on kiddie rides. And, if Emily's Bill didn't make rides safer for children, what was the point of passing it?

Then, to ratchet up the public pressure, Mike talked to *The Star* and *The News*. He gave voice to his outrage. "I'm not sure my family and I can in good conscience continue to support the bill. It flies in the face of what Emily's Bill was supposed to do—make rides safer for kids," he said. "This is ridiculous. We've got a bill that's necessary because a child got injured, my child, and the Senate wants to reduce the insurance limits for kids. Don't they know how offensive that is?"

His anger attracted public attention, but it didn't seem to be moving the Senate. A member of the Senate's Republican caucus called Mike and told him that the Republican caucus still couldn't support the higher insurance requirements. "We haven't got the votes, Mike," the senator said.

That meant that Mike had to go to the leadership—to Senate President Pro Tempore Bob Garton himself. Mike called Garton's office to get an appointment, and was told the senator was out. Mike left a message that was a thinly veiled threat. He said that he understood that Garton's caucus would not support increasing the insurance requirements and that he would like to talk with Senator Garton about that.

Translated, Mike's message meant that he was going to blame Garton if Emily's Bill failed to become law. Mike waited for a response to his message. It didn't come. It appeared that he had lost the game of chicken.

Mike's media barrage had, however, moved one person to action.

That person was Frank O'Bannon.

The governor called Mike to talk about the impasse, saying he thought it was really important to get Emily's Bill passed. Mike agreed, but argued that if the bill didn't require parks to carry more insurance, it would be essentially meaningless. All the work and sacrifice that went into the Emily's Bill struggle would have gone for naught.

Mike also pointed that the Senate's intransigence was silly, because representatives from the insurance industry had testified that they only wrote one million policies for amusement parks.

The governor listened, then asked Mike if he could be patient for a day or two. Mike said he could. O'Bannon signed off by saying that he would try to work something out.

Later, the governor called Luke Kenley. Frank O'Bannon and Luke Kenley had a lot in common. Both were soft-spoken men from small Indiana towns who liked to have people underestimate them. Each talked with a heavy Hoosier accent that stopped just short of sounding hayseed. Both were intensely bright and practical. And each knew that the art of politics involved timing—of knowing when to stand tough and when to cut a deal.

O'Bannon asked Kenley to get the Republican caucus to go along with the higher insurance numbers. The governor explained that the insurance industry already routinely required amusement parks to carry at least one million per accident. He said that it didn't make sense for the state and the Legislature to go through all the turmoil that had marked Emily's Bill without having something concrete to show for it.

Kenley listened, and agreed to go back to his caucus with the governor's message. He found the votes he needed.

On Monday, April 29, 1997, the House and the Senate voted on the final version of Emily's Bill. It passed the House 98-0. The Senate voted 38-9 in favor of it. Emily's Bill was on its way to the governor's desk. As soon as Frank O'Bannon signed it, it would become law.

After the deadlock broke, Mike sat down with Emily to tell her what had happened at the Legislature. He told her that Emily's Bill had cleared both houses of the General Assembly. She asked what that meant. He told her that it meant that Emily's Bill soon would be Emily's Rule and that it would make rides safer for children.

Emily kissed him on the cheek and said: "Thank you, Daddy. I'm so proud of you." Mike had experienced few better moments in his life.

CHAPTER EIGHTEEN

A LITTLE MORE THAN A WEEK AFTER THE INDIANA HOUSE OF Representatives and the Indiana Senate passed Emily's Bill, the Hunts and the Joneses loaded up their cars for another journey. This time, they went to the governor's office. They went to see Frank O'Bannon sign Emily's Bill into law.

It was a Thursday morning, May 8, 1997. The legislative session had ended tumultuously, with the Republicans in the House refusing to vote in favor of the budget. Their refusal meant that there would have to be a special session of the Legislature. The stakes for the special session were enormous. Whichever party seemed to win the budget battle would drive the state's agenda for perhaps the next two years. Both Republicans and Democrats were angry. The air around the State-house crackled with tension.

But not in the governor's office that morning. This Thursday morning in the governor's office, everyone in attendance seemed happy to be there—as if this moment represented the end of a long, hard journey.

In fact, the journey had been a hard one. At one time, Emily's Bill was the most divisive issue before the Indiana General Assembly. The acceptance of the minority committee report in the House had nearly produced a brawl. The maneuvering during the conference committee process had produced dissension in both caucuses of the Senate.

Many obstacles had barred the path for Emily's Bill's to becoming law. Most Statehouse observers had begun the session believing that even getting a hearing for the bill would be impossible. The disputes over the constitutionality of the original measure, the cost associated with paying Emily's medical bills and the entrenched and powerful interests lined up to oppose the bill seemed too formidable to be overcome. Somehow, though, Emily rolled over or past all of them.

During his trips to the Statehouse, Mike had discovered something. He had come to see the passage of Emily's Bill as a kind of spiritual gift. He felt that a greater force had guided him, and had moved aside the biggest barriers preventing Emily's Bill from becoming law. Although he knew that he had worked hard to get Emily's Bill passed, he didn't believe that his efforts had produced the victory.

He thought Emily had done that. It seemed to him that, at every difficult moment, his four-year-old daughter had reached out to strangers, both obscure and powerful, and reminded them of what was the right thing to do. Whenever Emily's Bill faced what seemed to be an insurmountable obstacle, Emily's story had touched someone, and the opposition melted away.

Emily had brought Governor O'Bannon around. She had brought Jesse Villalpando, John Gregg and the House of Representatives around. She had brought Luke Kenley and the Indiana Senate around.

It seemed as if people saw her picture—looked at her shy little girl's smile—and wanted to help her.

At one time, Emily's image had evoked something akin to pity. People looked at her, saw the wheelchair and felt sorry for her and her family. The long walk to pass Emily's Bill changed that. More and more, people came to think of Emily's story in another way—as proof that willing hearts and determined spirits could accomplish great deeds. Her courage told people that a hope could become a reality.

Frank O'Bannon understood that. In his press release announcing the signing of Emily's Bill, he spoke of Emily in glowing terms. "Out of this terrible tragedy that forever changed the life of a little girl comes something positive that will help prevent accidents like this in the future," the governor said in the press release.

"Emily's bill will not only make amusement parks safer. It will also provide more resources for families who, heaven forbid, face similar circumstances."

Then O'Bannon paid tribute specifically to Emily. "I thank Emily and her family for being here, and I salute her for her courage and spirit. Today's ceremony is in her honor, and the people of Indiana will forever be grateful to her and her dad for their dedication in pursuing this cause."

The language in the press release was exceedingly formal, almost arcane. The bill signing was decidedly less formal. The governor's office overflowed with TV cameras and newspaper reporters. Even though the office was a spacious one, it quickly came to seem cramped. People from all over the Statehouse had gathered to watch Emily's Bill become law.

Many of the familiar faces were there. Jesse Villalpando was there. So were Luke Kenley and Bill Alexa. They were all happy to be there. At a time when the mood in the Indiana General Assembly seemed to be turning increasingly ugly, this moment seemed especially joyful. It felt as if they had overcome turmoil and bitterness, avoided snares of partisanship and political rivalry, to finally come together and help a little girl. They felt as though they had accomplished something important and gathered around the governor's desk as Frank O'Bannon signed his name to House Bill 1431, and Emily's Bill became law.

One familiar face didn't show up for the signing: Candy Marendt decided not to go.

For her, the harsh feelings generated by the battle to get Emily's Bill out of the House still were too fresh and too unpleasant for her to overlook.

She knew that politicians were supposed to have tough

hides, that they were supposed to be able to forget things and move on once the jousting over a political issue was over, but the maneuvering over Emily's Bill had disgusted her. She had even been embarrassed about her own role in it. Candy had come to think of the speech she had made the night Emily went to the hospital and the House passed Emily's Bill as the worst of her life. She felt that she had let herself be drawn down into the muck, and that she had no one to blame but herself.

She knew that she had violated the rules of the House by directly impugning Jesse Villalpando's motives. She felt bad about that. Not long after the rancorous debate in the House over Emily's Bill, she tried to call Villalpando at his law office in Northern Indiana. She got his secretary, who asked Candy if she wanted to leave a message. Candy said that she hoped Representative Villalpando would call her back so she could apologize. That call never came.

Worse, she found that several Democrats whose friendship and opinion she valued now were reluctant to talk with her. They made it clear to her that they blamed her, not Jesse Villalpando, for the ugliness Emily's Bill had generated.

Candy knew that she hadn't tried to hijack the bill so she could ram one of her pet projects through the Senate. All she had tried to do was help a father whose family had suffered a horrible tragedy and who seemed to be in over his head at the Legislature. Somehow, she couldn't see how that made her the bad guy in the story.

Still, Candy didn't feel like attending the signing. Doing so would have meant standing next to Jesse Villalpando and smiling, and knowing all the while how much he still resented her and all she had done.

The important thing to Candy was that the bill had passed. Emily's medical bills would be paid. Amusement rides would be safer. She wanted to feel good about those things, and the way she had helped the Hunt family.

She wanted to take pride in the part she had played in making Indiana amusement parks more safe. Showing up at the signing wouldn't help her do that.

Mike Hunt felt a huge sense of relief when he watched Frank O'Bannon put his signature on Emily's Bill. Moments earlier, he, Amy and the girls had entered the office. Nikki, Emily's irrepressible twin sister, rushed right over to the big, comfortable chair behind the governor's desk. She sat down in it, and then began to spin it around, as if it were a toy that had been waiting just for her.

Seeing his daughter there lightened the mood, but only for a moment.

Mike could not help thinking about how difficult the climb since August had been. The months at the Legislature had been some of the hardest of Mike's life. In the early days of the session, he had slept hardly at all. Each night he had plotted and planned, convinced that any mistake or miscalculation he might make would further jeopardize his daughter's health and endanger his family's future.

As Mike watched the governor sign Emily's Bill, he thought about how much had changed.

He recalled those early weeks of frustration, when he had waited and pleaded for Frank O'Bannon to do something, anything, to show that he supported Emily's Bill. Mike remembered the gathering anxiety—the fear that almost approached panic—as he felt his chances of getting Emily's Bill heard were slipping away. It was hard at the time for Mike not to get angry with the governor, but it had been impossible for Mike to stay angry with Frank O'Bannon.

Even at the worst moments of the bill's bruising journey through the legislative process, Mike had retained his faith in the governor's basic decency. He always had believed that O'Bannon's word was good, that the governor was an honest man looking for an honorable and responsible way to keep his promise.

Now, Mike's faith had been rewarded.

Emily's Bill was law. Emily's medical expenses would be paid. The Hunt family had been saved from bankruptcy.

As Frank O'Bannon signed Emily's Bill into law, Mike sighed the sigh of a man who felt that he had narrowly averted a disaster.

The only sounds in the governor's office when Frank O'Bannon signed Emily's Bill came from the soft scratching of his pen on paper and the quiet hum of the TV cameras recording the moment. When the governor finished writing and stood up, the hush continued for a moment. Then, the small crowd applauded.

O'Bannon stood silent and smiled at those in attendance, a genial man radiating an avuncular charm.

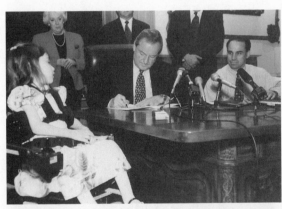

Emily and Mike look on as Governor Frank O'Bannon signs House bill 1431—Emily's Bill—into law.

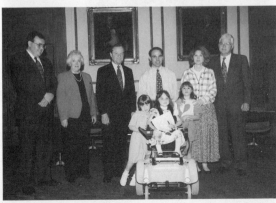

At the signing (l-r) Jesse Villalpando, Sue Landske, Frank O'Bannon, Mike, Amy and Bud stand behind Nikki, Emily and Sarah. Note Bud's and Amy's somber look.

Then he turned toward Emily, who was seated in her wheelchair just off to the governor's right. O'Bannon smiled at her. "I'll give you the pen," the governor told Emily. "It's not a very fancy pen, though." Emily smiled, and the crowd in the office laughed.

The governor said a few words about how Emily's Law would make amusement parks safer for the state's residents, particularly Indiana's children. He complimented Mike and Amy on their determination, and praised Emily's courage.

Then he asked Mike to speak. Mike kept his remarks simple. "This is his accomplishment," Mike said of O'Bannon. "He shows great concern for children."

Then Mike began to talk about what his struggle meant for the state of Indiana. He alluded to his early struggles to get the bill heard, to the forces that seemed to be aligned to defeat Emily's Bill because no powerful special interest stood behind it. He mentioned the great injustice that had been done to his family, to his little girl.

"This shows," Mike said, "that an ordinary guy can still come to the Statehouse and get justice." The passage of Emily's Bill showed, Mike said, that the system could work. With that, the formal portion of the bill signing ceremony ended. Normally, people are ushered out of a governor's office in a hurry. The crowd gathered in O'Bannon's office lingered. People chatted and shared memories. No member of the governor's staff urged them to leave, perhaps because everyone wanted to keep the good spirits generated by the moment alive for a little longer.

The governor himself knelt down so that he could talk face to face with Emily. He told her that she and her father had done a great thing for the state of Indiana.

Later, after the Hunts had gone home, Mike asked Emily what she thought of the ceremony in general and Governor O'Bannon in particular.

Emily thought for a moment before answering. "He's a real nice man," she said. "He's just like a grandpa."

CHAPTER NINETEEN

AFTER GOVERNOR O'BANNON SIGNED EMILY'S BILL INTO LAW, a lot of people wanted to congratulate Mike Hunt. They called him, wrote him, even stopped him on the street to say what a great thing it was that he had gotten Emily's Bill passed. They assumed that the bill's passage made him happy, and asked what he and his family had done to celebrate the "victory." They acted almost as if the battle to pass House Bill 1431 had been a football game and Mike had scored the winning touchdown. They seemed to be waiting for him to spike the ball in the end zone.

Mike knew most of these people were well meaning and that they were just trying to be kind to him and his family. At first, he tried to explain that the passage of Emily's Bill wasn't something his family would celebrate, that getting the bill passed was poor consolation for all that the family had lost. Having Emily's medical bills paid by the state did not compensate the family for not seeing their little girl run in her small skipping steps. And making amusements parks safer for people didn't begin to make up for losing Nancy.

When Mike tried to explain these things, though, all too often the eyes of the people he was talking to would go blank. He could tell that they didn't understand, and that they wanted to believe that Emily's Bill made for a happy ending, that the Hunt family was at peace, that all was right with them again.

It was more complicated than that. Ever since that August day when the kiddie train at Old Indiana jumped the tracks, change had battered the Hunts and the Joneses like the sheets of rain brought on by a gale. Every day brought a new challenge, new demands for courage, determination and compassion. From the moment that he first had heard about the wreck, Mike had lived in fear, afraid that he would fail, that his wife and his daughters would suffer even more because he hadn't been smart enough or tough enough or experienced enough to look out for them the way he should.

Even when he was on his way to the Statehouse to watch the governor sign Emily's Bill into law, he had felt a moment of terror. Panic seized him, and he began to wonder if he had just dreamed that Emily's Bill had passed both the House and the Senate. He wondered if he weren't still at the hospital, praying that Emily would live. *What if this is just a dream,* he thought, *and I wake up to find out that I still have this nightmare ahead of me?*

Once in the governor's office and at the bill-signing ceremony, he realized that Emily's Bill's passage was real, and he felt something else. Mike listened to the governor tell Emily in his aw-shucks Frank O'Bannon voice that he was proud to be part of making the bill law, and Mike felt overwhelmed by how powerful a thing love could be. Mike's whole body tingled at that moment. Without the love that his daughter inspired, his family still would be facing ruin. Still tingling, Mike silently thanked all of the people in the room. That tingle didn't last long.

Almost as soon as he finished with his thanks, Mike's thoughts turned to the one person in the family who couldn't be part of the bill-signing ceremony—his mother-in-law, Nancy.

There were some parts of the battle to get Emily's Bill passed that pleased Mike. He felt that he had learned a great deal. He felt that he understood suffering better than he had before, that dealing with his family's tragedy had unearthed depths of compassion in him that he hadn't known existed before the wreck. He thought he was more sensitive to others, and that he had a better, more humane understanding of what really matters in life. He believed that the accident had made him a better person, a better friend, a better husband, a better father. He was grateful for the growth; yet he knew that it had come at a dreadful cost, for the whole family. He could not help but feel that Nancy had paid the price for his personal enlightenment. That thought haunted him.

Mike wasn't the only member of the family to struggle with contradictory feelings at the bill-signing. Bud Jones attended the bill-signing, too. While the TV cameras focused on Emily, Mike and Amy, Bud stood silently off to the side. He didn't say a word, Couldn't say a word.

It took almost all of his self-control to control his rage. He still felt an anger that reached to his soul. Part of the ceremony seemed absurd to Bud. He couldn't understand why there had been such a huge fight over what seemed like such a simple idea—namely, that an amusement park for children ought to be a safe place. He thought that if the park's owners and the state had understood that from the beginning, he and his wife would be sitting down to dinner that night and his granddaughter Emily would come running up the driveway to give Nancy a hug on Saturday.

The day Emily's Bill was signed, Bud stood at the center of Indiana's state government, surrounded by family and other people who wished him well. He had rarely felt more alone in his life.

Bud's torment had not gone unnoticed. On the day of the signing, Bud stood next to Amy while the news photographers took pictures of the family posing with the governor. Amy heard her father sniffling. She looked over at him, and saw that there were tears in Bud's eyes.

After the photographers had finished and left, Amy looked over at her father again. His head was down. Ever since she was a little girl she had known that that was a sign that her dad was sad or depressed. His shoulders seemed to slump, and she knew then that he was thinking about her mother.

Without hearing a word from him, Amy knew just how lost and lonely her father felt.

The reason Amy could tell how much pain her father was in was because she felt it, too. The whole time she was in the governor's office she thought about her mother. A part of her still couldn't believe that Nancy wasn't there, that the whole tragedy was real. She wanted to think that her eyes would open and Emily would be walking again, holding Nancy's hand as they came back from a grandmother-granddaughter outing. Amy wished that Nancy could be there to hear the governor of the state tell Emily how brave she was.

Later, long after Emily's Bill had become law and he had stopped haunting the Statehouse, Mike finally figured out a way to explain the complicated set of feelings passing the bill aroused.

Imagine that you and your family fell into a deep pit, he would say. Somehow, you manage to start crawling upward. You dig and you scratch and you pull. You can even take some comfort from the fact that the climb has strengthened your muscles, and made you tougher than you were before. But you don't start celebrating until you climb all the way out. And you never forget the person you had to leave at the bottom of the pit.

CHAPTER TWENTY

Governor O'Bannon signed Emily's Bill into law on a spring day.

As spring blossomed into summer, Mike and the family settled into the slow march toward the first anniversary of the wreck and Nancy's death. The days were not empty. Now that the state had agreed to pay the bulk of Emily's medical bills and Emily's Bill had been passed, only one account remained to be settled.

Ever since the train derailed, the owners of the Old Indiana Family Fun-n-Water Park had done their best to avoid taking responsibility for the tragedy their negligence had brought about. Through their attorneys, they had skillfully parried Mike's attempts to attach liability to their carelessness by shifting blame onto the state and its inspectors. They had fought and beaten back Boone County Sheriff Ern Hudson's attempts to institute criminal proceedings against them.

Worse, in almost contemptuous defiance of public sentiment, they had even refused to apologize—to say that they were sorry that a woman had lost her life and a little girl had her spine broken because they couldn't be bothered to make their rides safe.

Mike and his attorneys searched for a way to make Old Indiana's owners accept some share of the blame for what had happened. Finally, they thought they had found that way.

The lawyers found that the park owners—Hagerman Construction, Steven Sohacki and his sons James and Reginald Sohacki—had declared bankruptcy three times. Each time they declared bankruptcy there had been some problem at the park. That history demonstrated a pattern of using bankruptcy to avoid taking responsibility for what they had done.

In early June, Mike sent a settlement offer to the lawyer representing the park's insurance company, a rather testy man named Bob Clemens, Mike gave the owners until August 11—the first anniversary of the wreck—for accepting the offer. Otherwise, he would file suit.

June, then July drifted by without a response. By August 11, neither the park nor its insurance company had responded, so Mike filed the suit. He knew that there wasn't much chance that he would win in court, but he wanted to make every attempt to hold the park's owners accountable for the damage they had done.

Once again, the Hunts were front-page news. The news accounts described the train derailment once more. There were brief recountings of the long march to get Emily's Bill passed. Then the stories took note of the fact that the state employees responsible for the wreck had been punished. The state itself had accepted responsibility for its part in the tragedy by agreeing to pay most of Emily's medical bills. Only one party to the accident still had not accepted any portion of the blame: the park's owners.

Clemens, the insurance company's attorney, exploded with anger. He complained to reporters that the Hunts were manipulating things. He even implied that the park's owners were the true victims, not the little girl in the wheelchair or her dead grandmother.

"If we try this case in the media," Clemens snarled, "I have no chance of winning it."

The suit was not the only milestone that summer. On June 29, Emily and Nikki turned 5. The family had a party, and everyone tried to be happy, but it was a bittersweet occasion—the first of Emily's birthdays Nancy had missed.

Bud tried to throw himself into caring for his children and grandchildren, but that wasn't necessarily an escape for him. Much of the joy he had taken from outings with his kids and grandkids came from the fact that the grandparents' weekends and parties were something he did with Nancy.

He could be particularly awkward around Emily. He loved her and would do anything for her, but seeing her only brought up memories of the wreck.

Mike and Amy did their best to prepare the girls for August 11. They told them that they were going to see where Grandma was buried so they could say goodbye to her. Mike thought it would be a good idea to lighten the mood by taking the children to see a movie, preferably a family-friendly comedy. He suggested that they go to *George of the Jungle*.

Emily grew hysterical. She screamed that she didn't want to go. Mike and Amy asked her why. The explanation came out between sobs. Emily had seen one of the TV commercials promoting the film, one in which George swings into a tree and everyone laughs.

"That's not funny," Emily said. "That how people die. That's how Grandma died." The Hunts didn't go to see the movie.

On August 11, Ern Hudson called Bud Jones at home. The two men had developed a friendship in the year since the accident. Ern told Bud that he was thinking about him, and that Bud and his family were in Ern's prayers. They talked for a while about how important family was, and then hung up. As Bud replaced the phone in its cradle, he found that he was crying.

The family gathered at Nancy's grave. They put flowers down and prayed. Everyone was quiet. Mike and Amy held hands and leaned on each other, each keeping an arm free for whichever child needed a hug.

Sarah grieved silently, but profoundly. She kept stealing glances at Bud to make sure he was all right.

Nikki had misunderstood Mike and Amy. She thought that they were actually going to see Nancy again at the gravesite, that she would be able to hug and talk to her grandmother again. When she learned the truth, the wound opened for her all over again. She began to wail, and could not be comforted.

Emily—G.G., "Grandmother's Goiter"—sat in her wheelchair, wept quietly and missed her grandmother.

The next day in the newspapers, Bob Clemens, the attorney for the Old Indiana Family Fun-n-Water Park's insurance company, issued a complaint.

He said that the Hunt family had treated his clients unfairly.

CHAPTER TWENTY ONE

WHEN EMILY HAD FIRST BEEN INJURED, MIKE AND AMY made the same assumption that almost all people do—that a spinal injury was irrevocable. That Emily had been condemned to a life of paralysis.

As they prepared for the long effort to pass Emily's Bill, though, they began to acquaint themselves with the research being done on spinal cord injuries. Their studies taught them something remarkable.

Not too many years before, an injury as severe as Emily's in a person as young as she was most likely would have been fatal. If a little girl with a severe spinal cord injury like Emily's had been able to survive, there was no chance that she ever would be able to walk again. Damaged spinal nerves couldn't be regenerated and the signals from the brain that traveled through the damaged area couldn't be rerouted. A person with a broken spine spent his or her life in a wheelchair. That was the best that could be hoped for. In recent years, however, researchers had made amazing breakthroughs.

They had discovered ways both to rejuvenate damaged spinal cord tissue and to reroute the communications from the brain stem. Their breakthroughs made it seem possible— even likely—that spinal cord injury victims soon would be able to leave their wheelchairs behind and walk again.

All they needed was money. The researchers estimated that spending an additional 300 million to 500 million dollars would result in a cure.

Once Mike learned that, he knew that he had to find a way to make a contribution. The best way he could contribute, he figured, was to raise money to fund the researchers who were working so hard to get his daughter out of the wheelchair. With his standard single-minded determination, Mike set about the task of raising as much money for spinal cord research as he could. He began organizing something he called Emily's Walk. It turned out to be bigger than even he could have imagined.

The first Emily's Walk took place on a lovely autumn day at the famed Indianapolis Motor Speedway, home of the Indianapolis 500. Thousands of people showed up. For weeks before the walk, families from all over Indiana had gone out with pledge cards, collecting promises from Hoosiers to lend their financial support to spinal cord research. It was a worthy cause, they told everyone they asked for money.

Even worthy causes can be too abstract for people to spend their time and their money on. A brave little girl in wheelchair was something else—a symbol of determination and courage that could touch almost anyone. That's what Emily did. Hoosiers had taken to her. In the words of her uncle, David Jones, it seemed as if the entire state wanted to adopt her.

When the crowd of thousands showed up at the Speedway that October day, they willingly dropped off their pledge cards, wrote their checks and handed over their cash. They knew that the reason that the Hunts had put together Emily's Walk was to raise money for research. That was their reason for turning out.

The crowd had another reason for showing up at Emily's Walk. They wanted to tell Emily and her parents how much they admired them and how much they cared about Emily. They wanted to tell the Hunts that they weren't alone. All day, people kept coming up to Emily and Mike and Amy to say how impressed they were with the way the family had responded to hardship and how much of an inspiration their struggle had been. All day, people from all around Indiana had been eager to shake Mike's hand or pat Emily on the head.

When the walk was over and all the pledges had been collected, Emily's Walk had raised more than $100,000. It was a record in Indiana for a first-time fundraising effort.

Not long after the first Emily's Walk, a group of out-of-state investors bought the Old Indiana Family Fun-n-Water Park from its owners. The new owners behaved more graciously than the old ones had. They exerted pressure on the old owners to arrive at a settlement with the Hunts so that the sale could go through.

After the sale was complete, the new owners said they planned to eventually reopen the park. They planned to rename it, though, out of respect for the people whose lives had been damaged at Old Indiana. They pledged to make safety their top priority.

Mike and Amy saw the new owners as angels, people who had come in to make certain that the right thing was done. They were grateful that the new owners had made the Hunts' satisfaction a priority.

Even so, one thing rankled. It still seemed as if the park's old owners had gotten away without admitting to any responsibility for the harm they had done.

The success of Emily's Walk prompted Mike to think bigger.

In the fall of 1997, he began putting together the Emily Hunt Foundation, a not-for-profit organization dedicated to finding a cure for spinal cord injuries. He put together a board of directors, more than a few of who had ties to the Emily's Bill struggle or to the development of Emily's Walk.

He and Bud and David were the first members of the board. Dr. Thomas Luerssen, Emily's doctor at Riley Children's Hospital also accepted a spot. So did two of the attorneys from Bingham Summers Welsh & Spillman, the law firm that had advised the Hunts ever since the wreck. Josie George, a member of the family that owned the Indianapolis Motor Speedway, took another board slot. She was particularly motivated, because her teen-age son had suffered a spinal cord injury. He had recovered. She wanted the same for all children.

It was an impressive group. Almost immediately, the board set forth an ambitious fundraising and public education program. They planned a series of events designed to make money for spinal cord research and tell people the day that people would be getting out of their wheelchairs was close.

The public education effort got a boost in January, 1998, when Frank O'Bannon gave his second State of the State address.

A year before at that time, Mike had just begun desperately working the halls of the Legislature, buttonholing the few members of the Indiana House of Representatives who would even deign to talk with him. Back then, he had sent note after note into the House for individual members to come out and chat for a minute about Emily's Bill. He had watched through the big picture windows at the back of the chamber as those notes were either ignored or thrown away. Back then, he had been fighting desperately just to get his foot in the door.

A year can make a huge difference.

For this State of the State, Mike and his family were honored guests of the governor. Mike, Amy, the girls and Bud showed up well before the speech. An escort from the governor's office took them upstairs to the House chamber. It was the first time any of them had set foot in the House.

They were brought to the front of the chamber, just a few feet away from the lectern where the governor would be delivering his speech. It was an almost bewildering moment for a family that had never expected nor wanted to do anything more than live their lives, do their work and raise their children. They wanted to be neighbors, not celebrities.

As the Hunts and the Joneses sat in front of the assembled House and Senate, Bud turned to Amy and said, "Can you believe this is happening?"

The governor began his speech by recounting the triumphs of the previous year. At the top of his list of his accomplishments was the passage of Emily's Bill, which he said would make Indiana's amusement parks much safer for children. O'Bannon said that the state had some people to thank for that achievement. He gestured toward where Mike, Amy, Emily, Nikki, Sarah and Bud sat. The TV cameras focused on the family. In their homes all across Indiana, Hoosiers watched Bud and the Hunt family as the governor paid tribute to them. The state owed Emily's Bill, O'Bannon said, to the courage of a little girl and the determination of her father to see that the right thing got done. The state, the governor said, owed Emily and Mike Hunt a big debt.

At that, all the members of the Indiana General—all the senators, all the representatives—leapt to their feet and gave a thunderous round of applause to the Hunts. A year can make a big difference.

The Emily Hunt Foundation grew almost astoundingly quickly. Within a year, it had raised almost a half-million dollars.

Some of the money came from a golf outing in the summer that Bud organized. Another $100,000 came from the second annual Emily's Walk at the Speedway. Still more came from a flurry of gifts during the year.

The highlight for the year, though, was undoubtedly the first Emily Hunt Gala, a black-tie dinner in downtown Indianapolis. The theme for the evening was Dreams of Dancing, a reference to Emily's ambition to be a ballerina. In her honor, a corps of ballet students donated their time to dance outside the ballroom where the gala was held while the guests filed in.

Many familiar faces showed up. The governor could not come because he had a schedule conflict. Candy Marendt showed up with her son in tow. Ern Hudson and Ken Campbell provided security for the event. The security was for the guest of honor, actor Christopher Reeve. Ever since Mike had begun to work the Statehouse to get Emily's Bill passed, events had conspired to bring him into contact with Reeve. The connection was a natural. After his injury in a horseback-riding accident, Reeve had become the most famous spinal cord injury victim in the world. He also had become America's leading activist in the field of spinal cord research. Once the Emily Hunt Foundation took flight, Mike had started to work more closely with Reeve.

Because of Mike's demonstrated fundraising ability, Reeve had agreed to come out to give a speech at the first Emily Hunt Gala. Reeve pulled in a crowd. More than five hundred people paid more than $100 a plate to hear him talk for twenty minutes.

The night seemed to have been conjured out of a spell. As a band played, the crowd danced. Mike and Amy danced, too. They gave themselves over to enjoying the good will people had for them. At one point, Bud came over to Emily's wheelchair and pretended to be reaching for her pony-tail. She gave a squeal of happiness.

When the program began, Reeve addressed the crowd from his wheelchair. He wore a dark blue sweater and casual slacks. He spoke slowly, in bursts of three, four or five words between the programmed breaths of the ventilator that he needed in order to stay alive. For much of the talk, the audience stood and paid rapt attention as Reeve told them that it was likely that Emily Hunt would walk again. He told them that they had it within their power to make it possible for people like him to get out of their wheelchairs.

When Reeve finished talking, the audience erupted in applause. It was a powerful talk, a moment alive with feeling. But it was not evening's most moving scene. That came after Reeve spoke.

As part of the gala's program, Mike planned to give the first Emily Hunt Award for courage to Matthew Ware, a local high school basketball player who had suffered a spinal cord injury while diving for a loose ball. While he was in the hospital, Ware and his family talked movingly of their faith—and of his determination to lead a meaningful life in spite of his injury.

Mike could think of no better person to receive the first Emily Hunt Award. The award was a gold medal. On the back of it, the words "With your courage you inspire others to achieve excellence" were inscribed.

Mike arranged things so that he could deliver a short talk in tribute to Ware's bravery and determination. When he finished talking, Emily was supposed to give Ware the medal. It almost worked that way. Mike spoke, briefly, movingly, about the strange twist of fate that had made him an unwilling public figure. He talked about the importance of supporting spinal cord research. He closed by saying that it gave him great pride to give a fine young man like Matt Ware the first award in his little girl's name.

When he finished speaking, Mike walked over to help Emily present the medal to Ware. As they tried to hand over the medal, it slipped out of their hands and fell to the ground. Mike immediately bent down to pick up the medal. At the same moment, Emily looked out at the crowd. She brought her hands up to her face and pressed them against her cheeks, almost as if in imitation of a silent film star saying, "Oh, no!"

The crowd's reaction came in waves. At first, everyone laughed. Then, the thought that it was almost miraculous that a little girl who had suffered so much could do something so winning, so funny, took hold of the audience. Everyone stood, and started to applaud. The applause went on and on.

Everyone wanted to give Emily and her family an ovation.

The crowd clapped and clapped and clapped for a little girl and her father who were making a long walk, a long walk from horror to hope.

EMILY AT NIGHT

WHEN THE SCHOOL DAY ENDS, GENERALLY AMY IS WAITING to take Emily and her sisters home. Once they get back to the house, Emily plows conscientiously into her homework. It comes quickly and easily to her. Most often, she's done in twenty minutes. When she's finished with her schoolwork, Emily has a snack and then spends some time having fun.

Some afternoons, she gets on her computer and plays games on the Internet. Some afternoons, she reads a mystery; she's particularly fond of Nancy Drew. Some afternoons, she parks herself in front of the television set and watches reruns of twenty-year-old game shows on Game Show Network. "My favorite is '$25,000 Pyramid,' " she says.

The entire family gathers for dinner around 6:30. At the table, the girls talk about their days at school. Emily often talks about how she and her friends were "walking" down the hall or on the playground when something happened to interest them.

Her parents gently quiz her about her word choice—*you were doing what?*

"I was walking with my friends," Emily continues.

You were what? Mike or Amy asks, teasing.

At that point, Emily gets it. She rolls her eyes, as if to say that she can't believe that her parents are being so literal.

"All right," she says, "I was rolling along in my chair beside my friends when...."

After dinner, Emily has a couple of hours to relax. She watches television or continues reading her mystery. When it's time for her to go to bed, her mother gets her ready.

Emily still remembers her grandmother. She remembers how she used to stay with Nancy. She remembers her grandmother's gentleness and how Nancy had a gift for making a shy little girl feel comfortable. "She was my favorite person," Emily says.

When Emily goes into her bedroom, her wheelchair rolls right by a little picture frame containing an embroidered message. It reads:

> *Some people come into our lives and quickly go ... some people stay for awhile and leave footprints on our hearts and we are never, ever the same.*

Once Amy has changed Emily into her pajamas and given her a good night kiss, it is time for Mike to come in.

He connects Emily to some oxygen so that she can breathe, and thus sleep, more deeply during the night. It goes into the tracheotomy tube in Emily's throat.

Being hooked to the oxygen means Emily cannot talk. Mike turns on a monitor, like a baby monitor, and tells Emily to make her "sound" if she needs anything. The sound is a clicking sound Emily makes with her tongue.

"You're okay. Click if you need me," Mike tells her before he kisses her good night. He knows that it is important for a little girl to feel safe and secure. He wants Emily to know that her father is watching out for her. The lights go out. Emily generally falls asleep quickly. And she dreams.

In her dreams, she's always walking. Sometimes, she's even dancing.

About the Author

John Krull has been the executive director of the Indiana Civil Liberties Union since July of 1998.

John came to the ICLU after a long career as a columnist, editorial board member, political reporter and feature writer for *The Indianapolis News* and *The Indianapolis Star.* In the seventeen years he spent at those two newspapers, his writing won more than three dozen journalism awards.

John lives in Indianapolis, Indiana, with his wife, the journalist Jenny Labalme, and their two small children, daughter Erin and son Ian.

Emily's Walk is his first book.

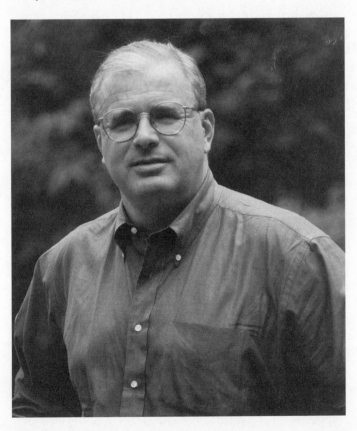

About the Emily Hunt Foundation

All of the royalties and sales proceeds from this book will benefit spinal cord injury research. The Emily Hunt Foundation, Inc., was formed on March 5, 1998. The mission of the organization is:

To seek a cure for people suffering from paralysis resulting from a spinal cord injury by raising funds to support scientific research, and increasing public awareness of the progress made in spinal cord injury research.

The Emily Hunt Foundation, Inc., is a not-for-profit corporation recognized by the Internal Revenue Service and the State of Indiana as a tax-exempt organization. Donations are fully tax deductible to the extent of the law. If you would like to make a donation, or want to know more about the Emily Hunt Foundation, you can contact us at:

The Emily Hunt Foundation, Inc.
PO Box 68093
Indianapolis, Indiana 46268
(317) 329-0805
www.emilywalk.com

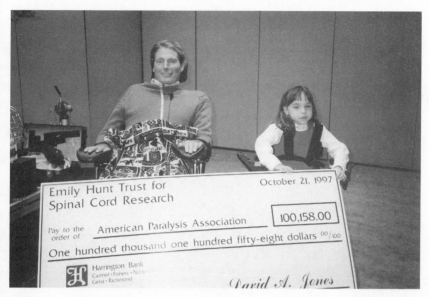

Emily meets actor Christopher Reeve for the first time to present him with a check for spinal cord research. These were the proceeds from the first Emily's Walk.

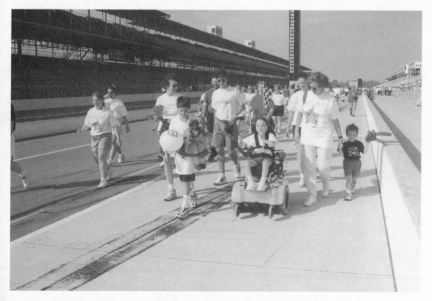

Emily leads the First Annual Emily's Walk for spinal cord research.